Pocket Atlas
of Radiographic Positi

Torsten B. Möller, M.D
Department of Radiology
Am Caritas Hospital
Dillingen, Germany

Emil Reif, M.D.
Department of Radiology
Am Caritas Hospital
Dillingen, Germany

In collaboration with

Dyan Attwood-Wood
Monika Braun
Beate Hoffmann
Sabine Figus
Hans Werner Oetjen
Christa Riegler

Translated by Horst N. Bertram

405 illustrations

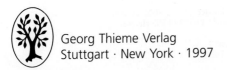

Georg Thieme Verlag
Stuttgart · New York · 1997

II

Library of Congress Cataloging-in-Publication Data

Möller, Torsten B.:
Pocket atlas of radiographic positioning / Torsten B. Möller ;
Emil Reif. In collab. with Dyan Attwood-Wood ... Tranl. by
Horst N. Bertram. – Stuttgart ; New York : Thieme, 1997
  Dt. Ausg. u. d. T.: Möller, Torsten B.: Taschenatlas Einstelltechnik
NE: Reif, Emil:

This book is an authorized translation of the German edition published and copyrighted 1995 by Georg Thieme Verlag, Stuttgart, Germany. Title of the German edition: Taschenatlas Einstelltechnik: Röntgendiagnostik, Angiographie, Computertomographie.

© 1997 Georg Thieme Verlag, Rüdigerstraße 14, D-70469 Stuttgart, Germany
Thieme Medical Publishers, Inc., 381 Park Avenue South, New York, NY 10016

Translated by Horst N. Bertram
Cover design by Dominique Loenicker

Typesetting by primustype Robert Hurler, D-73274 Notzingen
Printed in Germany by K. Grammlich, D-72124 Pliezhausen

ISBN 3-13-107441-8 (GTV, Stuttgart)
ISBN 0-86577-640-7 (TMP, New York)

For my brother Lars

Torsten Möller

For my sister Cornelia

Emil Reif

Preface

The subject of this book is radiographic imaging, the production of pictures of good quality as the diagnostic basis for the evaluation and interpretation of normal and abnormal, or pathological, anatomical findings. The arrangement of the material in this *Pocket Atlas of Radiographic Positioning* parallels closely that of the *Pocket Atlas of Radiographic Anatomy*, and, in some parts, that of the *Pocket Atlas of Cross-Sectional Anatomy*. This concurrent arrangement of contents should make it easy for the RT as well as the radiologically interested physician to cross-check and compare a correctly exposed radiographic view with normal anatomical findings.

There are many good books available on the subject. What was missing was a pocket book; a book that depicts—at a glance, distinctly and clearly arranged—all the important details that are needed for a good radiographic film; a book that, more than just clearly showing the ordinary, also informs about variations and offers practical "Tips & Tricks"; a book that presents, at one glance, all the criteria of a well-exposed radiographic view.

To accomplish these objectives, well over 200 ink drawings were required –; drawings, because these can be reduced to essentials and thus enable the "quick glance." The two-color design of the pictures also added to their comprehensibility. Details such as projection, central ray, or cassette position are easily seen.

For added clarity, the text is systematically structured into paragraphs describing (1) imaging parameters, (2) positioning and technique, and (3) variations. "Tips & Tricks," where appropriate, are presented separately, as are the "Criteria of a Good Radiographic View," which are demonstrated on original X-ray pictures. This way, too, the attention of the less-experienced reader is directed to the essentials.

We are particularly pleased that we were able to enlist the cooperation of some of the best RTs from different institutions for our project. Their contributions to this book ensure that there is no undue emphasis on "in-house" techniques and that these techniques and their variations are applicable anywhere. Also included were Anglo-American radiographic approaches and techniques to ensure universal applicability. Without a doubt, the fruitful and detailed discussions of many questions also added to the quality and usefulness of this book as a teaching manual for the training of technologists and to its value for use in daily practice.

Extensive collaboration of this kind has been unique in the field, and we therefore wish to express our sincere thanks to Dyan Attwood-Wood, Monika Braun, Beate Hoffmann, Sabine Figus, Michaela Knittel, Sabine Mattil, Christa Riegler, Brigitte Schild, Claudia Zimmer, and Hans

Werner Oetjen. Sincere thanks are also due to Drs. Markus Bach, Horst Bertram, Albert Schmitt, Patrick Rosar, Wolfgang Theobald, Stephan Knittel, Beate Hilpert, Ute Marquardt, and to the RTs of our practice for their friendly and knowledgeable critique and advice. And thanks, too, to my mother, Friedel Möller, for her support and advice regarding the artistic layout.

Dillingen, August 1996   Torsten B. Möller and Emil Reif

Addresses

Dyan Attwood-Wood
Head MTRA
Institute of Clinical Radiology
Westf. Wilhelm University of Münster
48149 Münster, Germany

Monika Braun
Head MTRA
Department of Radiology
Am Caritas Hospital
66763 Dillingen/Saar, Germany

Beate Hoffmann
Head MTRA
LETTE-MTA-Training Institute
Viktoria-Luise-Platz 6
10777 Berlin, Germany

Sabine Figus
Klinikum Ludwigshafen
MTA Training Institute
Bremserstraße 79
67063 Ludwigshafen, Germany

Torsten B. Möller, M.D.
Department of Radiology
Am Caritas Hospital
66763 Dillingen/Saar, Germany

Hans Werner Oetjen
Head MTRA
Editor, *Radiologie-Assistent*
Am Ring 7
25917 Stadum, Germany

Emil Reif, M.D.
Department of Radiology
Am Caritas Hospital
66763 Dillingen/Saar, Germany

Christa Riegler
Head MTRA
Department of Radiology
Städtisches Krankenhaus
71065 Sindelfingen, Germany

Contents

Skull

Spine

Upper Extremity

Lower Extremity

Other Non-Contrast Diagnostic Studies

Gastrointestinal Examinations

Intravenous Examinations

Angiographies

Computed Tomographies

Skeletal Diagnosis

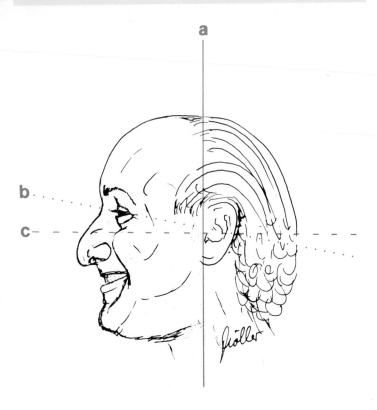

a Vertical auricular line (connects both external auditory meatus, divides skull into two halves)

b Eye–ear line (orbitomeatal line, extends from the outer canthus of the orbit to the external auditory meatus)

c Horizontal infraorbitomeatal line (from the bony inferior orbital rim to the external auditory meatus)

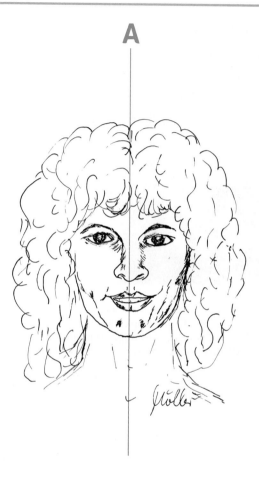

A = Median line

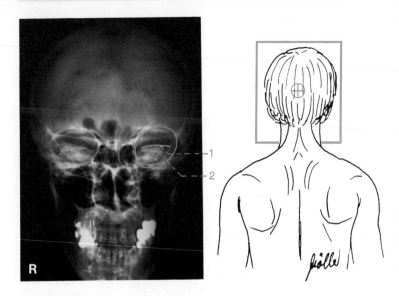

■ **Criteria of a Good Radiographic View**
— Skull symmetrical and completely visualized
— Skull PA: superior petrous ridge (1) projects into midorbit (2)
— Skull AP: superior petrous ridge projects into the lower third of the orbit
— Outer table of the skull visible

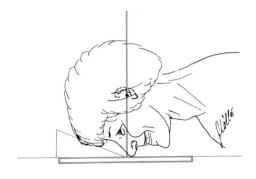

Imaging Technique
Film size: 10 × 12" (24 × 30 cm), lengthwise
Film speed: 200
FFD: 40" (115 cm)
Bucky: yes (under the table)
Focal spot: large
Exposure: 70–75 kV, automatic, center cell

Patient Preparation
— Remove dentures, glasses; open braids
— Remove jewelry (necklace, earrings, hairpins, glasses, hearing aid)
— Open clothes (buttons, zipper)

Positioning

— Prone, arms along sides of the body
— Forehead supported on a sponge wedge, tip of the nose rests on the
 table, chin is flexed (horizontal infraorbitomeatal line is vertical)
— Supine position, head flexed so that the horizontal infraorbi-
 tomeatal line is vertical, support the head if necessary
— Tilt tube to align the central ray parallel to the horizontal infraorbi-
 tomeatal line, median plane in middle of the film, skull straight
— Head immobilized with weighted band
— Skull filter, "keyhole," long portion over the region of the cervical
 spine
— Gonads shielded (large lead apron)

Alignment
— Projection: (1) PA, or (2) AP, perpendicular to the film at the middle
 of the skull
— Central ray directd to occipital protuberance at the center of the
 film
— Centering and collimation, side identification
— No breathing or swallowing during the exposure

Tips & Tricks
The skull is straight when both auditory meatus are projected at the
same level.

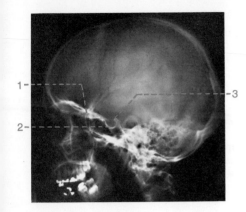

■ **Criteria of a Good Radiographic View**
— Complete visualization of the entire skull
— Both temperomandibular joints superimposed
— Lesser and greater sphenoid wings of both sides superimposed (1)
— Sella linear (2) (no double line)
— Clinoid processes superimposed (3)

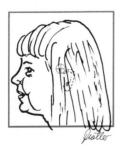

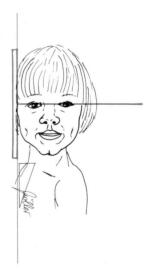

Imaging Technique
Film size: 10 × 12" (24 × 30 cm), crosswise
Film speed: 200
FFD: 40" (115 cm)
Bucky: yes (under the table)
Focal spot: small
Exposure: 65–70 kV, automatic, center cell

Patient Preparation
— Remove dentures, glasses, hearing aids, etc.
— Remove jewelry (necklace, earrings, hairpins)
— Open clothes (buttons, zipper)

Positioning

— Prone (or seated), side of the skull to be examined adjacent to the film
— Upper arm along the side of the body, forearm rests on the table
— Anterior shoulder and chin supported with sponge wedge so that the median plane of the skull is parallel to the film
— Upper border of the cassette 2 FB above the skin line (or simply: middle of the cassette = middle of the skull)
— Skull immobilized with weighted band
— Skull filter
— Gonads shielded (long lead apron)

Alignment
— Projection: lateral, perpendicular to the film
— Central ray directed to the middle of the skull (about 1 cm above and in front of the external auditory meatus, center of the film)
— Centering and collimation, side identification
— No breathing or swallowing during the exposure

Tips & Tricks
Put a pillow wedge under the chest of thin patients and children so that the median sagittal plane of the skull is parallel to the table.

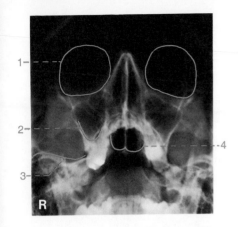

■ **Criteria of a Good Radiographic View**
— Both orbits symmetrical (1)
— Superior petrous ridges (3) below antral floors (2)
— Sphenoid sinus (4) projected through the open mouth

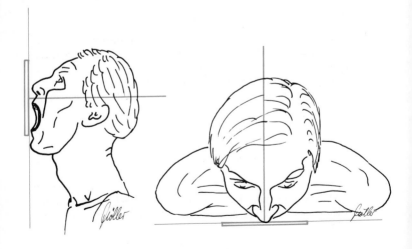

Imaging Technique
Film size: 5 × 7" (13 × 18 cm) or 10 × 12" (24 × 30 cm), lengthwise
Film speed: 200
FFD: 40" (115 cm)
Bucky: yes (under the table)
Focal spot: small/large
Exposure: 77 kV, automatic, center cell

Patient Preparation
— Remove dentures, glasses; open braids
— Remove jewelry (necklace, earrings, hairpins)
— Open clothes (buttons, zipper)

Positioning
— Facing the film (seated erect)
— Head straight (median sagittal plane perpendicular to the table)
— Head extended backwards so that the chin touches and the tip of the nose is about 1 FB from the vertical cassette
— Mouth wide open
— Gonads shielded (lead apron)

Alignment
— Projection: occipitonasal
— Central ray enters 2 FB above occipital protuberance, emerges at the level of the upper lip (directed at maxillary antrum or inferior orbital rim) in the center of the film
— Centering and collimation, side identification
— No breathing or swallowing during the exposure

Tips & Tricks
— Before taking the exposure, tape a paper towel to the cassette holder to put chin and mouth against (hygiene)
— If the patient cannot extend the head far enough, have him or her rest it on chin and nose, move the tube cephalad and angle the central ray correspondingly, craniocaudad (mostly 12°, but possibly up to 30°)
— The cross in the center of the upright bucky may be used as a centering aid: center of the cross directly below the nose

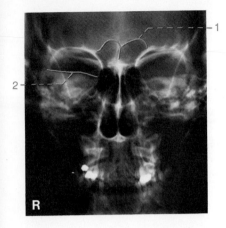

■ **Criteria of a Good Radiographic View**
  — Frontal sinuses completely visualized (1)
  — Both superior petrous ridges (2) projected over the upper orbital third

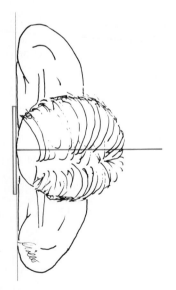
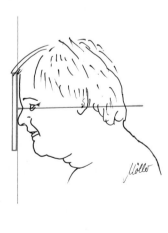

Imaging Technique
Film size: 5 × 7" (13 × 18 cm) or 8 × 10" (18 × 24 cm), lenghtwise
Film speed: 200
FFD: 40" (115 cm)
Bucky: yes (under the table)
Focal spot: large
Exposure: 77 kV, automatic, center cell

Patient Preparation
— Remove dentures, glasses; open braids
— Remove jewelry (necklace, earrings, hairpins)
— Open clothes (buttons, zipper)

Positioning

— Facing the film (sitting upright, hands used for support)
— Head straight (median sagittal plane of the skull perpendicular to the film)
— Forehead and tip of the nose resting against the cassette
— Possible use of extension cone
— Gonads shielded (long lead apron)

Alignment
— Projection: occipitonasal, perpendicular to the film
— Central ray directed to the nasion in the center of the film
— Centering and collimation, side identification
— No breathing or swallowing during the exposure

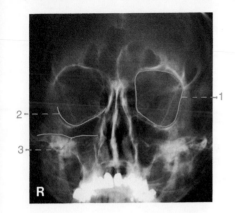

■ **Criteria of a Good Radiographic View**
— Symmetrical projection of both orbits without superimposition (1)
— Both superior petrous ridges (3) projected below the orbital floors (2)

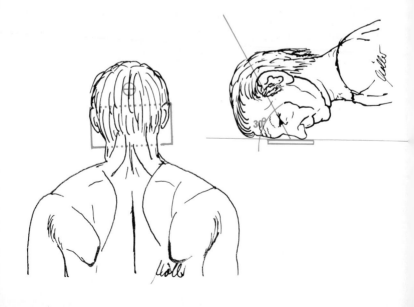

Imaging Technique
Film size: 8 × 10" (18 × 24 cm) – 5 × 7" (13 × 18 cm), crosswise
Film speed: 200
FFD: 40" (115 cm)
Bucky: yes (under the table)
Focal spot: small
Exposure: 70 kV, automatic, center cell

Patient Preparation
— Remove dentures, glasses; open braids
— Remove jewelry (necklace, earrings, hairpins)
— Open clothes (buttons, zipper)

Positioning

— Facing the film, prone position, arms along the sides of the body
— Head straight (exactly median), resting on forehead and tip of the nose
— Gonads shielded (lead apron)

Alignment
— Projection: occipitonasal, 30° craniocaudad
— Central ray (directed through the median plane to the occiput and nasion in the center of the film
— Centering and collimation, side identification
— No breathing or swallowing during the exposure

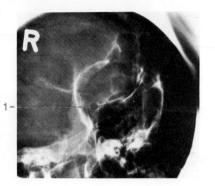

1 –

Criteria of a Good Radiographic View
Optic foramen (1) projected clearly into the lower outer quadrant of the orbit

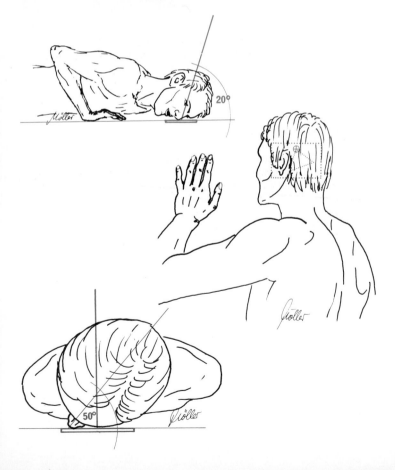

Imaging Technique
Film size: 5 × 7" (13 × 18 cm), crosswise
Film speed: 200
FFD: 40" (115 cm)
Bucky: yes (under the table)
Focal spot: small/large
Exposure: 70–77 kV, automatic, center cell

Patient Preparation
— Remove dentures, glasses; open braids
— Remove jewelry (necklace, earrings, hairpins)
— Open clothes (buttons, zipper)

Positioning

— Facing the film (sitting or prone position)
— Tip of the nose and zygomatic arch of the side to be examined resting against the cassette (face turned 50° to the exposed side)
— Orbit in the center of the film
— Gonads shielded (lead apron)

Alignment
— Projection: occipito-orbital, 5°–15° craniocaudad
— Central ray enters at the vertex of an equilateral triangle whose baseline connects the mandibular angle (mastoid process) to the occipital protuberance
— Central ray emerges in the middle of the orbit
— Centering and collimation, side identification
— No breathing or swallowing during the exposure

Tips & Tricks
Always take both sides for comparison.

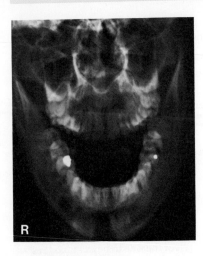

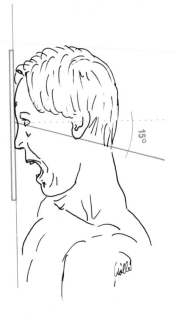

■ **Criteria of a Good Radiographic View**
— Complete visualization of the lower jaw
— Symmetrical projection of the temporo – mandibular joints

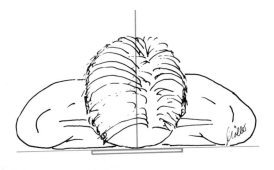

Imaging Technique
Film size: 8 × 10" (18 × 24 cm), lengthwise
Film speed: 200
FFD: 40" (115 cm)
Bucky: yes (under the table)
Focal spot: small
Exposure: 66–73 kV, automatic, center cell

Patient Preparation
— Remove dentures, glasses
— Remove jewelry (necklace, earrings, hairpins)
— Open clothes (buttons, zipper)

Positioning

— A. Patient seated erect (cervical and thoracic spine extended) in front of the upright cassette stand, head straight, chin flexed, forehead and nose resting against the cassette, mouth opened wide
— B. Prone position, forehead and nose resting against the cassette with mouth closed, then mouth opened wide for the exposure
— Gonads shielded (lead apron)

Alignment
— Projection: occipitomental, 15° caudocranial
— Central ray directed to the nasion
— Centering and collimation, side identification
— No breathing or swallowing during the exposure

Tips & Tricks
— Use a cork to help hold the mouth open
— In the prone position, put a low sponge wedge under the thorax

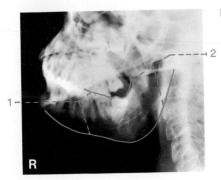

Criteria of a Good Radiographic View

— Horizontal (1) and vertical (2) portions of the mandible are shown free of overlying shadows

— the side of the mandible away from the film and the cervical spine are not superimposed

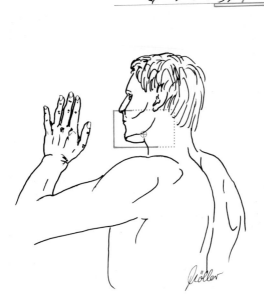

Imaging Technique

Film size: 8 × 10" (18 × 24 cm), crosswise   Film speed: 200
FFD: 40" (100–115 cm)   Bucky: no (yes)   Focal spot: small
Manual exposure: 57 kV; 25 mAs,   …mAs,   …mAs,   m..mAs
(with bucky 66 kV, automatic, center cell)

Patient Preparation

— Remove dentures, glasses, jewelry (necklace, earrings, hairpins)
— Open clothes (buttons, zipper)

Positioning

— Prone position, or patient seated obliquely in front of the upright
  cassette stand, head turned sideways, temple of the side to be examined resting against the cassette (median plane of the head at an
  acute angle to the stand = the mandibular ramus away from the film
  is projected cephalad out of view), chin pushed forward (to project
  the mandible away from the spine)
— Gonads shielded (large lead apron)

Alignment

— Projection: lateral, 25° caudocephalad
— Central ray 1 FB below the mandibular angle of the distant side,
  directed to the middle of the affected mandibular ramus
— Centering and collimation, side identification
— No breathing or swallowing during the exposure

Variations

1. Mandibular condyles, Schuller position: p. 33
2. Mandibular condyles, Parma position:
    — Head true lateral, median plane parallel to the cassette, affected side
      placed adjacent to the cassette
    — Projection: lateral, 5° caudocephalad
    — Central ray 2–3 FB anterior to the external auditory meatus,
      directed to the upper lip and to the TMJ adjacent to the film, mouth
      as wide open as possible
3. — Patient seated with the affected side toward the vertical bucky grid
    — Head tilted toward the stand, temple and zygoma resting against
      the vertical cassette
    — Central ray through the center of the mandibular ramus adjacent to
      the film (5 cm below the distant mandibular angle)
    — Projection: vertical or 10° caudocephalad

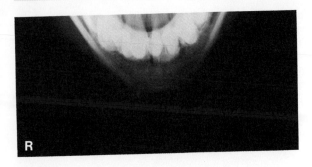

■ **Criteria of a Good Radiographic View**
Symmetrical view of chin and lower front teeth

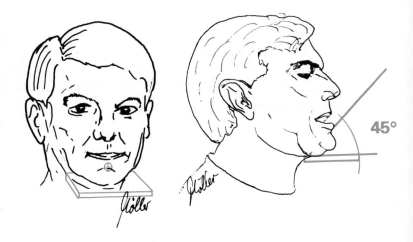

45°

Imaging Technique
Film size: 8 × 10" (18 × 24 cm), crosswise
Film speed: 200
FFD: 40" (100 cm)
Bucky: no
Focal spot: small
Manual exposure: 50–55 kV; 20–25 mAs,   …mAs,   …mAs,
…mAs

Patient Preparation
— Remove dentures

Positioning

— Patient sits in front of the examining table
— Cassette raised to chin level (put on a wooden box or patient's adjustable stool lowered)
— Patient extends chin forward as far as possible and rests it parallel to
  the film in the middle of the cassette (median sagittal plane of the
  head perpendicular to the film)
— Gonads shielded (large lead apron)

Alignment
— Projection: oblique, 45°, from cranioventral to causodorsal (supe-
  rior anterior to inferior posterior)
— Central ray directed in median plane through the lower lip
— Centering and collimation, side identification
— No breathing or swallowing during the exposure

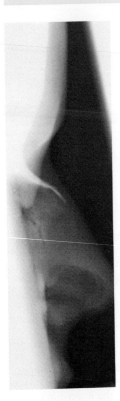

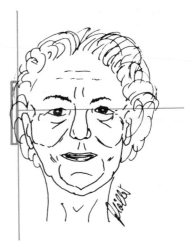

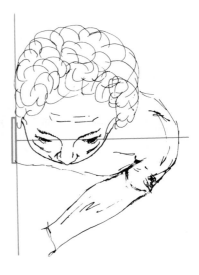

■ **Criteria of a Good Radiographic View**
Nasal bones including anterior nasal spine in straight lateral projection

Imaging Technique
Film size: 8 × 10" (13 × 18 cm), crosswise
Film speed: 100
FFD: 40" (100 cm)
Bucky: no (tabletop exposure)
Focal spot: small
Manual exposure: 44 kV; 12 mAs,   …mAs,   …mAs,   …mAs

Patient Preparation
— Remove glasses and jewelry

Positioning

— Patient sits with side to the upright cassette stand or lies recumbent
  in prone or supine position
— Head positioned straight lateral adjacent to the cassette (median
  sagittal plane of the skull parallel to the film)
— Gonads shielded (long lead apron)

Alignment
— Projection: lateral, perpendicular to the film
— Central ray directed to the nasion
— Centering, collimation to the tip of the nose

Variation
Film taken in supine position, head straight, cassette upright on edge

Tips & Tricks
When the film is taken with the patient sitting up, use a head clamp
to immobilize the occiput.

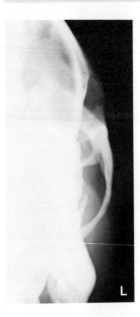

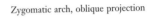
Zygomatic arch, oblique projection

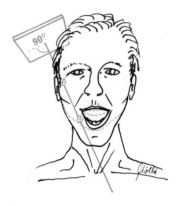

■ **Criteria of a Good Radiographic View**
Zygomatic arch projected without any superimposed structures

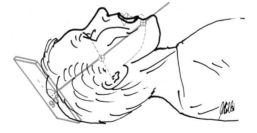

Imaging Technique
Film size: 8 × 10" (13 × 18 cm), lengthwise
Film speed: 100
FFD: 40" (100 cm)
Bucky: no (tabletop exposure)
Focal spot: small
Manual exposure: 60 kV; 25 mAs,   …mAs,   …mAs,   …mAs

Patient Preparation
— Remove dentures, glasses
— Remove jewelry (necklace, earrings, hairpins)
— Open clothes (buttons, zipper)

Positioning
— Supine, arms along the sides of the body
— Head straight, chin slightly extended
— Mouth closed while directing the central ray, opened wide for the exposure
— Head immobilized with weighted band
— Gonads shielded (large lead apron)
— After setting up the projection, cassette is placed behind the head, perpendicular to the central ray, upright and immobilized (with a sandbag or wedge)

Alignment
— Projection: oblique, from ventral–caudal–medial to dorsal–cranial–lateral
— Central ray directed along a line from the middle of the zygomatic arch to the anterior border of the mandible (at the level of the pre-molar of the adjacent side)
— Centering and collimation, side identification
— No breathing or swallowing, mouth opened wide during the exposure

Tips & Tricks
Middle of the zygomatic arch = midpoint between outer canthus and external auditory meatus.

Zygomatic Arch (continued from p. 25)

Variation

"Henkeltopf" ("jug handle") view (for comparison of zygomatic arches)

— Supine position, head overextended (shoulders supported on sponge pad)
— Projection: submentovertical (ventro-occipital, AP) at 45° angle to the horizontal infraorbitomeatal line
— Central ray 4 cm below mental symphysis (with mouth closed, mouth then opened wide for the exposure), transverse centering through the middle of the zygomatic arch
— Cassette parallel to the X-ray tube and perpendicular to the median plane, behind the head (see above)
  Tips and tricks. If there is soft-tissue swelling over the zygomatic region, turn the head slightly toward the swelling.

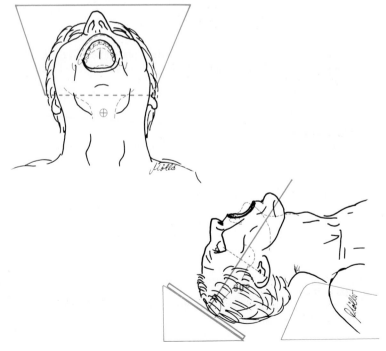

"Henkeltopf" "jug handle" view

Imaging Technique

Film size: 10 × 12" (24 × 30 cm), 8 × 10" (18 × 24 cm), lenghtwise
Film speed: 200
FFD: 40" (115 cm)
Bucky: yes (under the table)
Focal spot: large
Exposure: 77 kV, automatic, center cell

Patient Preparation

— Remove dentures, glasses; open braids
— Remove jewelry (necklace, earrings, hairpins)
— Open clothes (buttons, zipper)

Positioning

— Supine, arms along sides of the body
— Head straight, chin in maximal flexion, head supported with small wedge (orbitomeatal line perpendicular to the table)
— Mouth closed
— Head immobilized with weighted band
— Gonads shielded (lead apron)
— Adjust cassette to central ray (upper cassette border: 3 cm below skin border)

Alignment

— Projection: AP (vertico-occipital)
— Towne: 30° craniocaudad
— Altschul–Uffenforde: 35° craniocaudad
— Central ray directed to hairline (passing through external auditory meatus) and to the foramen magnum, or somewhat above
— Centering and collimation (especially Altschul), side identification
— No breathing or swallowing during the exposure

Variation

Vertico-occipital projection of the occiput, as in Towne position, but 45° craniocaudad angulation

(continued on pp. 28, 29)

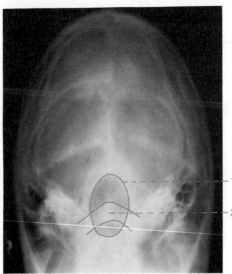

Towne position

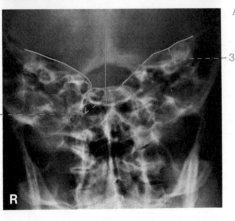

Altschul position

Criteria of a Good Radiographic View

Towne
— Symmetrical, clear view of the occiput (1)
— Posterior arch of atlas (2) projected over the foramen magnum

Altschul–Uffenforde
— Petrous bones and internal auditory canals (3) overlying the orbits
— Symmetrical projection, i. e., tips of the petrous pyramids (4) equidistant to the inner tables of the lateral calvaria

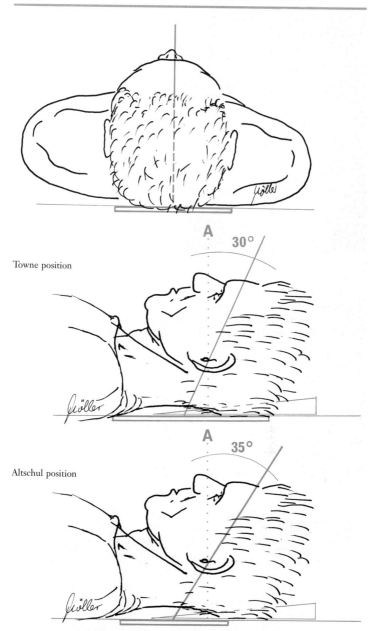

A

30°

Towne position

A

35°

Altschul position

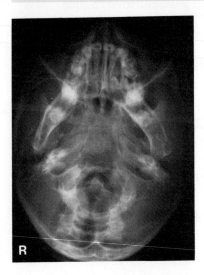

■ **Criteria of a Good Radiographic View**
  — Symmetrical base of the skull
  — Mandible projected over frontal sinuses
  — Symmetrical view of the mandibular condyles
  — Foramen ovale and spinosum are demonstrated

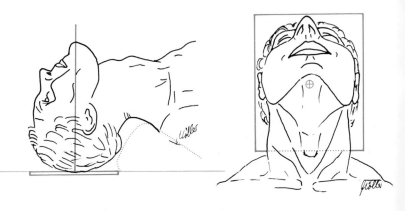

Imaging Technique
Film size: 10 × 12" (24 × 30 cm), lengthwise
Film speed: 200
FFD: 40" (115–100 cm)
Bucky: yes (no)
Focal spot: large
Exposure: 77 kV, automatic, center cell

Patient Preparation
— Remove dentures, glasses
— Remove jewelry (necklace, earrings, hairpins)
— Open clothes (buttons, zipper)

Positioning

— Supine position, either shoulders and back supported (elevated), or patient placed at the end of the bucky table
— Head extended far back so that vertex rests on the film
— Gonads shielded (lead apron)

Alignment
— Projection: axial, submentovertical
— Central ray directed to the floor of the mouth at the level of the external auditory meatus, perpendicular to the horizontal infraorbitomeatal line (inferior orbital rim – upper margin of the external auditory meatus)
— If the head cannot be sufficiently extended, compensate by tilting the tube
— Centering and collimation, side identification
— No breathing or swallowing during the exposure

Tips & Tricks
— All preparations, including getting the equipment and cassette ready, should be completed before positioning the patient, since the hyperextension of the head is very uncomfortable; after the film has been taken, the head should be lifted up immediately with both hands and put in a comfortable position
— Extend the head so far back that the shadow of the tip of the nose is projected on the cassette

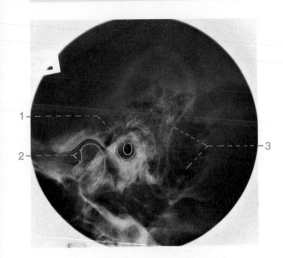

▦ Criteria of a Good Radiographic View
— External and internal auditory meatus (1) superimposed as perfectly round openings
— Mandibular condyle and joint fossa sharply defined (2)
— Complete visualization of the mastoid cells (3)

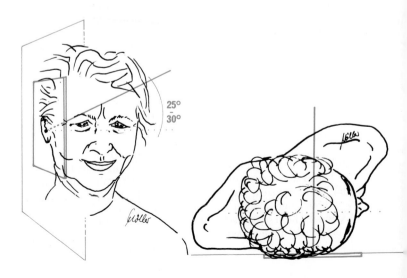

25° – 30°

Imaging Technique
Film size: 8 × 10" (13 × 18 cm), lengthwise/crosswise
Film speed: 200
FFD: 40" (115 cm)
Bucky: yes
Focal spot: small
Exposure: 77 kV, automatic, center cell

Patient Preparation
— Remove dentures, glasses
— Remove jewelry (necklace, earrings, hairpins)

Positioning
— Prone (or anterior oblique) position, side of the skull to be examined adjacent to the film; arm along the side of the body, forearm on the table for support; chin depressed so that the horizontal infraorbitomeatal line is perpendicular to the long axis of the table; anterior shoulder and chin elevated with a wedge until median sagittal plane of the skull is parallel to the film
— The auricle adjacent to the film is folded anteriorly to clearly show the mastoid cells
— Mouth wide open (to demonstrate the tips of the petrous pyramids)
— External auditory meatus of the side adjacent to the film at the center of the cassette, according to the oblique projection
— Head immobilized with weighted band
— May require use of extension cone
— Gonads shielded (large lead apron)

Alignment
— Projection: lateral, 30° craniocaudad
— Central ray directed to the auditory meatus of the side to be examined (4 FB above the auditory meatus of the healthy side), and middle of the film
— Centering, side identification (for recumbent position)
— No breathing or swallowing during the exposure

Variation
— Schuller technique for the demonstration of the temporomandibular joints
— Schuller variations:
  Rundstrom projection I—15° tilt instead of 30° (Henschen projection)
  Rundstrom projection II—35° tilt instead of 30° (Lysholm projection)

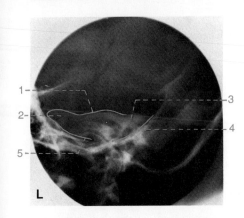

■ **Criteria of a Good Radiographic View**
— Petrous apices (2) clearly demonstrated
— Crista occipitalis interna (4) lateral to the superior semicircular canal (3)
— Superior petrous ridge horizontal (1)
— Inferior petrous ridge well demarcated (5)

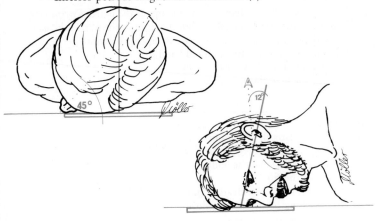

Tips & Tricks
When positioning the patient, one must watch that the median plane is not tilted. It is therefore best to turn the patient's head from a straight lateral into a 45° position.

Imaging Technique

Film size: 8 × 10" (13 × 18 cm), crosswise
Film speed: 200
FFD: 40" (115 cm)
Bucky: yes
Focal spot: small
Exposure: 65 kV, automatic, center cell (or manual 65–70 kV; 80 mAs, …mAs, …mAs)

Patient Preparation

— Remove dentures, glasses; open braids
— Remove jewelry (necklace, earrings, hairpins)
— Open clothes (buttons, zipper)

Positioning

Prone position
— Arms along the sides of the body
— Cervical spine straight, chin flexed (orbitomeatal line perpendicular to the film)
— Head turned 45° to the healthy side (supported with sponge wedge) = zygomatic arch and tip of the nose
Supine position
— Head turned 45° to the healthy side, chin flexed until horizontal infraorbitomeatal line (line A) is perpendicular to the top of the table
— Head immobilized with weighted band (pillow support)
— Gonads shielded

Alignment

Prone position
— Projection: oblique, 12° craniocaudad
— Central ray directed to the midpoint of a line connecting the external occipital protuberance and the mastoid process (about 2 FB medial and 2 FB caudal to the protuberance), transverse centering through the external auditory meatus of the side adjacent to the film
Supine position
— Projection: oblique, 12° craniocaudad
— Central ray from the midpoint of the orbitomeatal line 1 FB towards the orbit
— Centering, collimation, side identification (identify side to be examined, reverse mirror view)
— No breathing or swallowing during the exposure

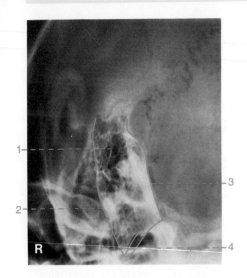

- **Criteria of a Good Radiographic View**
  — Complete visualization of the petrous bone (along its long axis) from the mastoid cells (1) to the apex (4)
  — Long axial projection of the anterior (2) and posterior (3) surfaces
  — Structures of the inner ear well exposed

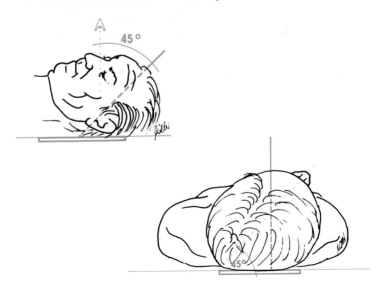

Imaging Technique
Film size: 8 × 10" (13 × 18 cm), lengthwise
Film speed: 200
FFD: 40" (115 cm)
Bucky: yes (under the table)
Focal spot: large
Exposure: 77 kV, automatic, center cell

Patient Preparation
— Remove dentures, glasses
— Remove jewelry (necklace, earrings, hairpins)
— Open clothes (buttons, zipper)

Positioning

— Supine, arms along sides of the body, chin depressed
— Head turned 45° to the side to be examined (supported with sponge wedge)
— Head immobilized with weighted band
— Gonads shielded (lead apron)

Alignment
— Projection: oblique, 45° craniocaudad angulation to the horizontal infraorbitomeatal line (A)
— Central ray directed to the hairline at the level of the lateral orbital border (frontal eminence of the distant side directed towards the mastoid process adjacent to the film)
— Centering and collimation, side identification
— No breathing or swallowing during the exposure

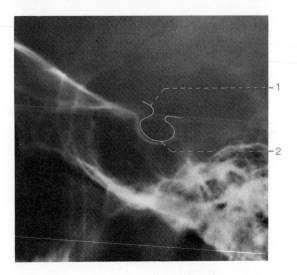

■ **Criteria of a Good Radiographic View**
— Sella, single contour (no double line) (2)
— Clinoid processes superimposed (1)

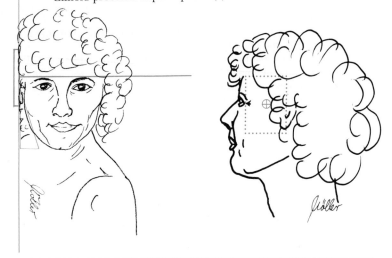

Tips & Tricks
If a lateral skull film was taken, take a film of the sella from the other side, in opposite projection.

Imaging Technique
Film size: 8 × 10" (13 × 18 cm), crosswise
Film speed: 200
FFD: 40" (115 cm)
Bucky: yes (under the table)
Focal spot: small
Exposure: 65–70 kV, automatic, center cell

Patient Preparation
— Remove jewelry (necklace, earrings, hairpins); take off glasses

Positioning

— Prone (or sitting), head straight lateral, adjacent to the film
— Arm along the side of the body, forearm resting on the table
— Anterior shoulder and chin elevated with a wedge pillow so that the median sagittal plane of the skull is parallel to the plane of the film (back of the head also supported with a sponge)
— Head immobilized with weighted headband
— Use an extension cone (for a "spot film")
— Gonads shielded (long lead apron)

Alignment
— Projection: lateral, perpendicular to the film
— Central ray directed to the midpoint of a line that connects the upper corner of the auricle with the outer canthus (2.5 cm above and anterior to the external auditory meatus) in the middle of the film
— Centering, collimation (not smaller than field size), side identification

Variation
Sella: PA projection
— 8 × 10" (13 × 18 cm), lengthwise; 77 kV; otherwise as above
— Prone position, head rests on forehead, chin slightly flexed, tip of the nose just touches the table
— Projection: vertical, occipitofrontal (PA)
— Central ray directed to the occiput, exits at the root of the nose (nasion), at the middle of the cassette
— Close collimation

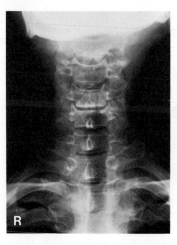

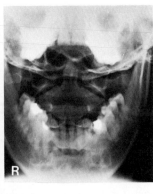

Criteria of a Good Radiographic View

— Odontoid process, axis and atlas are clearly visible through the open mouth, occiput does not obscure the odontoid, atlantoaxial and atlanto-occipital articulations are clearly defined
— Cervical vertebrae 3–7 clearly visualized, superior and inferior vertebral plates linear

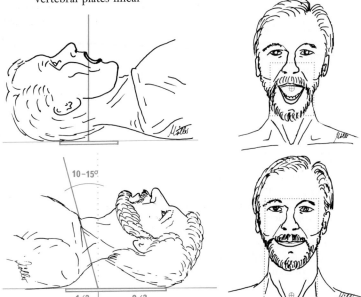

Imaging Technique
Film size: 8 × 10" (13 × 18 cm) (odontoid), 18 × 24 cm (cervical spine), lengthwise
Film speed: 200
FFD: 40" (115 cm)
Bucky: yes
Focal spot: small
Exposure: 65 kV, automatic, center cell

Patient Preparation
— Remove dentures, glasses
— Remove jewelry (necklace, earrings, hairpins)
— Open clothes (buttons, zipper)

Positioning

— Supine position
Atlas and odontoid process, AP
— Head flexed until upper teeth (occlusal plane) and occipital bone are superimposed (head elevated 15° with sponge wedge)
— Mouth wide open
Cervical spine, AP
— Head reclined so that the line of the mental symphysis – lower border of the occipital bone (imaginary line: corner of the mouth –auditory meatus) is perpendicular to the horizontal plane of the film
— Mouth closed
— Gonads shielded (lead apron)

Alignment
Atlas and odontoid process of the axis, AP
— Projection: ventrodorsal, perpendicular to the film
— Central ray in midline at the level of the corners of the mouth
Cervical spine, AP
— Projection: 10–15° craniocaudad
— Central ray directed to the sternal notch and middle of the cassette
— Centering and collimation, side identification

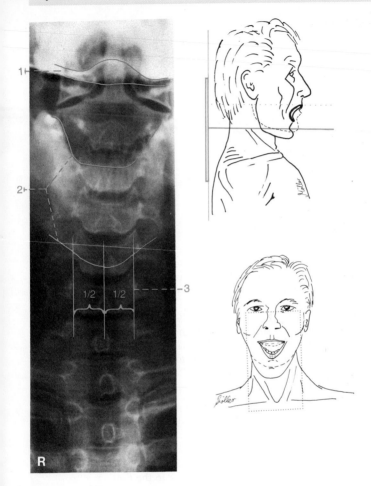

■ **Criteria of a Good Radiographic View**
— Symmetrical visualization of all 7 cervical vertebrae
— Occiput and maxilla superimposed (1)
— Lower jaw is blurred out (2)
— Spinous processes in midline (3)

Imaging Technique

Film size: 8 × 10" (18 × 24 cm), 10 × 12" (24 × 30 cm), lengthwise
Film speed: 200
FFD: 40" (115 cm)
Bucky: yes (under the table)
Focal spot: small
Exposure: 55 kV, automatic, center cell
Exposure time at least 3 seconds

Patient Preparation

— Remove dentures, glasses
— Remove jewelry (necklace, earrings, hairpins)
— Open clothes (buttons, zipper)

Positioning

— Patient sits with his back to the upright cassette stand
— Chin flexed (line connecting the occipital protuberance – occlusal plane of the maxilla is horizontal)
— When ordered "mouth open–closed, open–closed," patient moves only the lower jaw
— However, head must be held still (headclamp on forehead)
— Upper border of the cassette 1 FB below the corners of the eyes
— Gonads shielded

Alignment

— Projection: ventrodorsal (AP), perpendicular to the film
— Central ray directed to the chin (with mouth closed)
— Centering and collimation, side identification
— Patients may breathe while opening and closing their mouths during the exposure

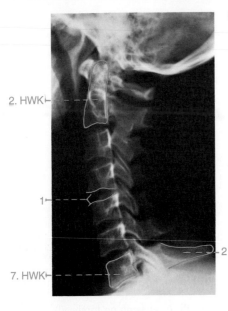

2. HWK

1

7. HWK

2

■ **Criteria of a Good Radiographic View**
— All 7 cervical vertebrae in straight lateral projection
— Straight projection of superior and inferior plates (especially 4th cervical vertebra) (1)
— Spinous process of the 7th cervical vertebra completely included (2)

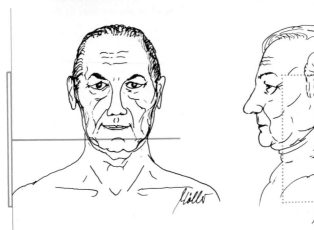

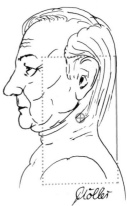

Imaging Technique
Film size: 10 × 12" (24 × 30 cm), (8 × 10", 18 × 24 cm), lengthwise
Film speed: 200
FFD: 40" (115 cm)
Bucky: yes (under the table)
Focal spot: small
Exposure: 60–70 kV, automatic, center cell

Patient Preparation
— Remove dentures, take off glasses
— Remove jewelry (necklace, earrings, hairpins)
— Open clothes (buttons, zipper)

Positioning

— Patient sitting erect, shoulder towards the upright cassette stand
— Head and neck straight lateral (median plane parallel to the film)
— Weights in both hands to pull the shoulders down
— Chin slightly lifted (so that the mandible is not superimposed on the cervical spine)
— Upper cassette border 3 cm above corner of the eye (8 × 10" cassette at canthus level)
— Gonads shielded

Alignment
— Projection: lateral, perpendicular to the film
— Central ray directed to the middle of the neck (4th cervical vertebra) and middle of the cassette
— Centering (orbit outside the radiographic field), collimation, side identification
— Breath held after expiration

Variation
— Magnifying view of the cervical spine: like cervical spine, but FFD only 32" (80 cm)
— Median plane (nose) at mid-distance between film and focal point (at 40 cm)

Tips & Tricks
Longitudinal centering along the midline of the neck (photocell likewise positioned over the middle of the neck).

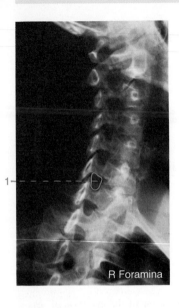

R Foramina

Criteria of a Good Radiographic View
Intervertebral foramina clearly demonstrated (1)

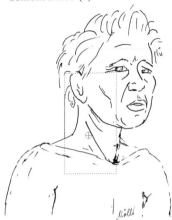

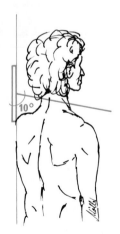

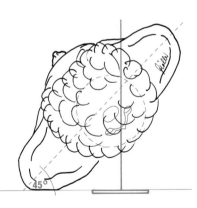

Imaging Technique

Film size: 10 × 12" (24 × 30 cm), 8 × 10" (18 × 24 cm), lengthwise
Film speed: 200
FFD: 40" (115 cm)
Bucky: yes (under the table)
Focal spot: small
Exposure: 60–70 kV, automatic, center cell

Patient Preparation

— Remove dentures
— Remove jewelry (necklace, earrings, hairpins)
— Open clothes (buttons, zipper)
— Hair (braid) combed up or to the side

Positioning

— Patient seated erect, with the back to the upright cassette stand
— One side of the back turned 45° away from the cassette
— Weights in both hands (sandbags) to pull the shoulders down
— Chin slightly lifted (head may be turned slightly towards the plane of the film to get the ramus of the mandible out of the picture)
— Upper border of the cassette = 3 cm above upper border of the ear
— Gonads shielded (small lead apron)

Alignment

— Projection: ventrodorsal (AP), 10° caudocephalad
— Central ray directed to the middle of the neck (4th cervical vertebra) and middle of the cassette
— Centering and collimation, side identification
— Breath held after expiration

Tips & Tricks

Magnifying view of the cervical spine: like regular oblique cervical spine, only:
— FFD 32" (80 cm)
— Median plane (nose) at mid-distance between film and focal point (at about 40 cm)
Side identification: left shoulder towards the stand = right foramina
right shoulder towards the stand = left foramina

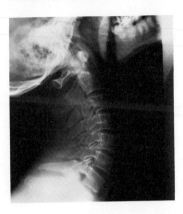 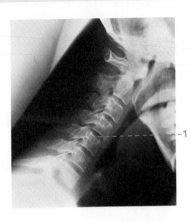

■ **Criteria of a Good Radiographic View**
— Straight lateral projection of the inferior and superior plates of the 4th cervical vertebra (1)
— All 7 cervical vertebrae are shown in maximal flexion and extension

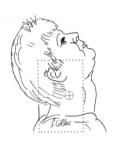 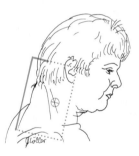

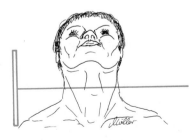 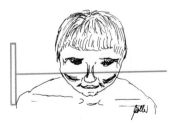

Imaging Technique

Film size: 10 × 12" (24 × 30 cm), lengthwise (extension) and crosswise (flexion)
Film speed: 200
FFD: 40" (115 cm)
Bucky: yes (under the table)
Focal spot: small
Exposure: 65 kV, automatic, center cell

Patient Preparation

— Remove dentures
— Remove jewelry (necklace, earrings, hairpins)
— Open clothes (buttons, zipper)

Positioning

— Patient seated erect, shoulder straight lateral to the vertical cassette stand
— Head and neck straight lateral, median plane parallel to the plane of the film
— Weights (sandbags) in both hands to pull down the shoulders (shoulder area may have to be immobilized)
— Head in maximal flexion and extension
— Longitudinal centering (and photocell) adjusted accordingly
— Lower cassette border 3 FB below vertebra prominens (7th cervical vertebra)
— Gonads shielded

Alignment

— Projection: lateral, perpendicular to the film
— Central ray directed to the middle of the neck (4th cervical vertebra) and middle of the cassette
— Centering, collimation, mark the side adjacent to the film
— Breath held after expiration
— One view each in maximal flexion and extension

Tips & Tricks

— Centering (and photocell) over the middle of the neck
— Always label the films
— to immobilize the head in flexion, use a head clamp for the forehead; in extension, use one for the back of the head

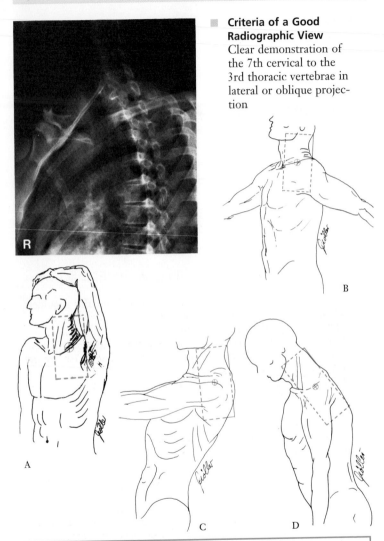

Criteria of a Good Radiographic View
Clear demonstration of the 7th cervical to the 3rd thoracic vertebrae in lateral or oblique projection

A

B

C

D

Alignment
— Projection: lateral or oblique, perpendicular to the film
— Central ray directed to the middle of the cassette
— Centering, collimation, side identification
— Breath held after expiration

Imaging Technique
Film size: 8 × 10" (18 × 24 cm), lengthwise
Film speed: 200 -/+ (+ for the thoracic spine)
FFD: 40" (115 cm)
Bucky: yes (under the table)
Focal spot: small
Exposure: 60–70 kV, automatic, center cell

Patient Preparation
— Remove dentures
— Remove jewelry (necklace, earrings, hairpins)
— Open clothes (buttons, zipper)

Positioning

A. Oblique
— Patient stands upright with the back to the film, distant side turned 20° away from the vertical cassette stand
— The arm away from the film is lifted up, the arm close to the film hangs loosely
B. Oblique
— Patient stands upright with one side against the vertical stand
— Arm close to the film is extended forward, the other arm backward
— Have the patient turn the side of the body that is away from the film back (about 20°) so that the humeral heads are not superimposed
C. Lateral ("waterskiing position")
— Patient stands straight lateral before the vertical bucky tray stand
— Patient bends the upper body back (dorsiflexion of the lumbar spine)
— Arms are extended forward (holding on to something in front)
— (Examination can also be done sitting down: both hands grasp the flexed knees and pull the shoulders forward)
D. Lateral (bending forward)
— Patient stands straight lateral before the vertical bucky tray stand
— Patient bends forward with straight back until the head, which is also inclined forward, rests against the headrest
— Both shoulders and arms are dropped forward and down, arms straight and turned inward (hands clasped between thighs)
— Upper border of the cassette 2 FB above the 7th cervical vertebra
— Longitudinal centering: (B–D) 3 FB anterior to the spinous processes, (A) through the anterior axillary line of the side away from the film
— Gonads shielded

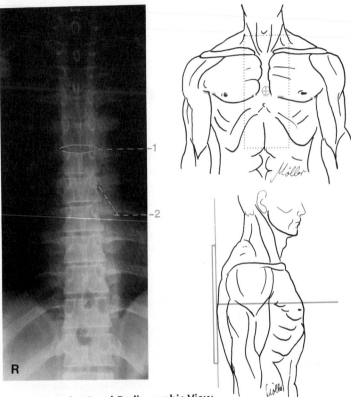

R

Criteria of a Good Radiographic View
— Well-exposed view of all thoracic vertebrae, including cervicothoracic and thoracolumbar junctions, well-demonstrated intervertebral spaces
— Superior and inferior vertebral surfaces clearly delineated (1)
— Costal junctions sharply defined (2)

Tips & Tricks
— Compensating filter instead of screen
— Centering aid: thoracic inlet (sternal notch) and midepigastrium (solar plexus) palpated with both hands, center = midway between both
— In the supine position, a small bag with rice flour may be placed over the cervicothoracic junction of the spine
— If there is a marked kyphosis present, decrease the focal film distance (more nearly parallel projection due to greater divergence of the beam)

Imaging Technique
Film size: 7 × 17" (18 × 43 cm), (20 × 40 cm), lengthwise
Film speed: 200 (400), compensating screen –/+
FFD: 40" (115 cm)
Bucky: yes (under the table)
Focal spot: large
Exposure: 75–85 kV, automatic, center cell

Patient Preparation
— Remove jewelry (necklace)
— Tie braid on top of the head
— Remove clothes from the waist up
— Remove shoes

Positioning
— Patient stands with the back to the cassette stand, arms hang along sides
— Legs are parallel, chin lifted
— Compression band over the lower chest
— Upper border of the cassette at the level of the 6th cervical vertebra (2 FB above 7th vertebra (vertica prominens), 1 FB above superior shoulder margin
— Gonads shielded

Alignment
— Projection: ventrodorsal (AP)
— Central ray directed to the middle of the sternum and middle of the cassette
— Centering and collimation, side identification
— Breath held after expiration

Variations
Films taken in supine position
— Legs drawn up, otherwise as above
Thoracolumbar junction
— Film size: 8 × 10" (18 × 24 cm), lengthwise
— Film speed: 200 (400)
— Central ray 1–2 FB below xiphoid process, in midline
— Films taken in supine position (legs drawn up)
— Otherwise as above

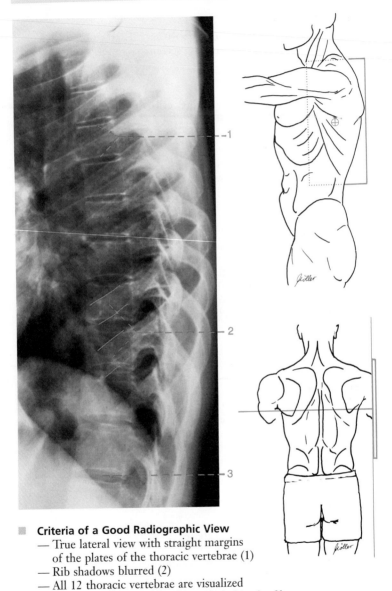

■ **Criteria of a Good Radiographic View**
— True lateral view with straight margins
   of the plates of the thoracic vertebrae (1)
— Rib shadows blurred (2)
— All 12 thoracic vertebrae are visualized
— Thorocolumbar junction (3) included in the film

Imaging Technique
Film size: 7 × 17" (18 × 43 cm) (20 × 40 cm), lengthwise
Film speed: 200 (400), compensating screen + – +
FFD: 40" (115 cm)
Bucky: yes (under the table)
Focal spot: large
Exposure: 85 kV, automatic, center cell

Patient Preparation
— Remove jewelry (necklace)
— Remove clothes from the waist up, take off shoes

Positioning

— Patient stands with the shoulder towards the cassette stand
— Both legs parallel
— Arms extended forward (holder support) or extended up above the head (patient grasps elbows)
— Upper border of the cassette at the level of the 6th cervical vertebra (2 FB above vertica prominens) or of the 7th vertebra (vertica prominens)
— Gonads shielded

Alignment
— Projection: lateral
— Central ray (a) one hand's breadth anterior to the posterior border of the skin and (b) at the level of the inferior angle of the scapula, directed to the middle of the cassette
— Centering and collimation, side adjacent to the film identified
— No suspension of breathing, have patient "continue to breathe quietly" during the exposure (ribs are blurred)

Variation
Films taken supine
— Exposure with breathing suspended (to prevent motion on the film)
— Knees flexed, otherwise as above
Thoracolumbar junction, lateral projection:
like recumbent technique, only:
— Film size: 8 × 10" (18 × 24 cm), lengthwise
— Central ray directed 1–2 FB below the xiphoid, and 4 FB anterior to the spinous processes

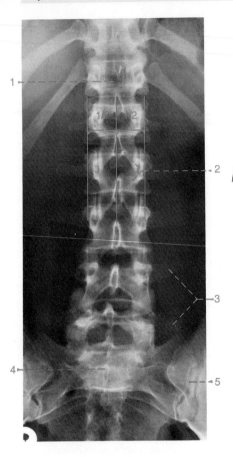

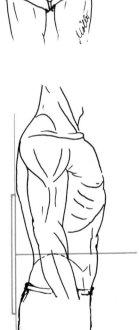

■ **Criteria of a Good Radiographic View**

— Entire lumbar spine, including T12 (1) and S1 (4), is on the film
— Spinous processes in midline (2)
— Sacroiliac joints (5) and transverse processes (3) are visible
— On films taken supine: straight projection of the margins of the plates of the lumbar vertebrae

Imaging Technique
Film size: 7 × 17" (18 × 43 cm) (20 × 40 cm), lengthwise
Film speed: 400 (200, 600)
FFD: 40" (115 cm) (–150 cm)
Bucky: yes (under the table)
Focal spot: large
Exposure: 75–85 kV, automatic, center cell

Patient Preparation
— Remove all clothes except undergarments
— Remove shoes

Positioning

— Patient stands with the back to the cassette stand, arms hang down
— Legs straight and parallel (if legs are of unequal length, support and build up the shorter leg, and note on the film)
— Compression band across the abdomen
— Middle of the cassette 2 FB above the iliac crest (L4)
— Gonads shielded (testicle cups for men, small lead apron for women, who hold the apron themselves)

Alignment
— Projection: ventrodorsal (AP), perpendicular to the film
— Central ray directed to the middle of the cassette
— Centering and collimation (not too close because of the sacroiliac joints), side identification
— Breath held after expiration

Variation
Lumbar spine, AP, supine
— Supine position, legs slightly flexed to reduce the lumbar lordosis, feet set on the table, otherwise as above
Lumbosacral junction, AP projection
— Supine position, hips and knees strongly flexed, feet on the table, thighs slightly abducted
— Film size: 8 × 10" (18 × 24 cm), lengthwise
— Central ray: 3–4 FB below the iliac crest in midline
— Tube may be angled 20° caudocephalad (Barsony technique)

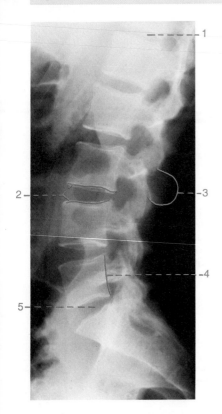

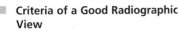

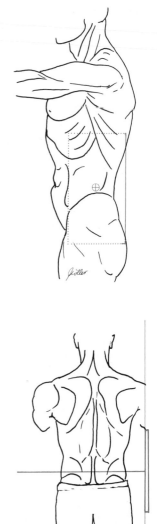

■ **Criteria of a Good Radiographic
View**
— True lateral view with straight
projetion of the plates of the
lumbar vertebral bodies (around
the central ray at L3/L4) (2)
— Thoracolumbar (1) and lumbosacral (5) junction well demonstrated
— Spinous processes well visualized (3)
— Posterior border of the vertebral
body linear in contour (4)

Tips & Tricks
If there is a marked levoscoliosis present, turn left shoulder towards
the cassette stand.

Imaging Technique
Film size: 7 × 17" (18 × 43 cm) (20 × 40 cm), lengthwise
Film speed: 400, –/+ compensating screen
FFD: 40" (115 cm) (150 cm)
Bucky: yes (under the table)
Focal spot: large
Exposure: 90 kV, automatic, center cell

Patient Preparation
— Remove all clothes except undergarments (take off shoes)

Positioning

— Patient stands with the right shoulder (lateral) towards the cassette
stand
— Legs straight and parallel, feet slightly spread
— Arms extended forward (holder support) or extended above the
head
— Middle of the cassette 2–3 FB above the level of the iliac crest (L3/
L4)
— Gonads shielded for males

Alignment
— Projection: lateral, perpendicular to the film
— Central ray (a) 2–3 FB above iliac crest, (b) one hand's breadth ante-
rior to the posterior skin border (about midpoint of a line extending
from the anterior superior iliac spine to the posterior border of the
sacrum, in the middle of the cassette
— Centering and collimation, side adjacent to the film identified
— Breath held after expiration

Variations
Films taken supine
— Legs pulled up (to reduce lordosis), patient put on padding to prevent
"sagging" of the lumbar spine (lumbar longitudinal axis), sponge
placed between the knees and parallel to the table top to prevent tilting
Lumbar junction, lateral projection
— Transverse centering about 3 FB below pelvic crest, otherwise as above

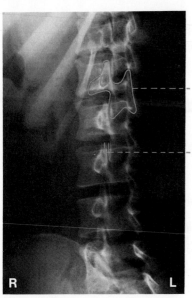

Criteria of a Good Radiographic View
— All 5 lumbar vertebrae show the "Scottie dog" sign (1)
— Intervertebral (apophysial) joints clearly demarcated (2)

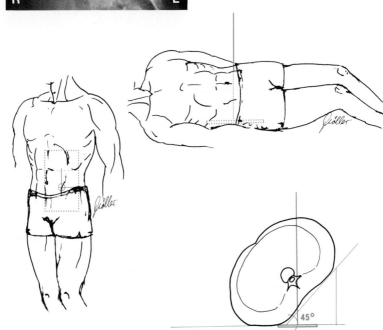

45°

Imaging Technique
Film size: 7 × 17" (20 × 40 cm), lengthwise
Film speed: 400 (200) (possibly compensating screen
+/– FFD: 40" (115 cm)
Bucky: yes (under the table)
Focal spot: large
Exposure: 80–90 kV, automatic, center cell

Patient Preparation
— Remove all clothes, except undergarments

Positioning

— Supine oblique, about 45° (more than 35°, not quite 45°) rotation
— Placed on sponge wedges (one under shoulder blades and one under sacrum to turn the upper trunk into an oblique position)
— Spine extended, legs drawn up to reduce lordosis (knees supported)
— Elevated side of the body straight (median plane parallel to the longitudinal axis of the body)
— Arms extended forward or above the head
— Middle of the cassette 2 FB above pelvic crest (slightly above umbilicus)
— Gonads shielded (for males)

Alignment
— Projection: oblique ventrodorsal (AP), perpendicular to the cassette
— Central ray (a) 2 FB above pelvic crest and (b) 2 cm medial (towards the umbilicus) of the anterior superior iliac spine of the elevated side (directed to the midpoint of a line from the last rib to the tip of the sternum)
— Centering and collimation, sides marked (R and L to indicate adjacent side of the body and intervertebral [apophysial] joints)
— Breath held after expiration

Tips & Tricks
For a marked lordosis: adjust the projection 15° caudocephalad.

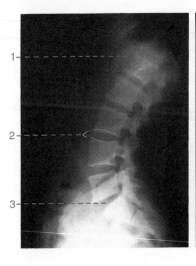
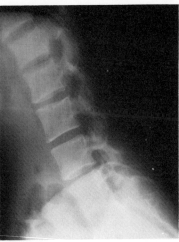

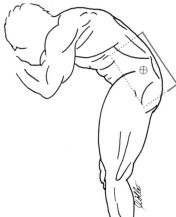
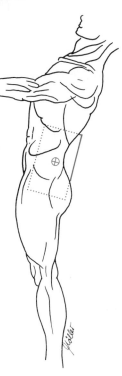

■ **Criteria of a Good
Radiographic View**
— True lateral projection, plates
of the vertebral bodies
straight (2)
— Visualization of all 5 lumbar
vertebrae, and of the thoracolumbar (1) and lumbosacral
(3) junctions

Imaging Technique
Film size: 7 × 17" (18 × 43 cm) (20 × 40 cm), lengthwise
Film speed: 400, compensating screen +/– FFD: 40" (115 cm)
Bucky: yes (under the table)
Focal spot: large
Exposure: 90 kV, automatic, center cell

Patient Preparation
— Remove all clothes except undergarments
— Remove shoes

Positioning

— Patient stands straight lateral to the cassette stand
— Legs straight and parallel, feet slightly spread
— Arms extended forward (holder support) or forward over the head
— Maximal flexion and extension
— Middle of the cassette 2 FB above pelvic crest
— Gonads shielded for males

Alignment
— Projection: lateral, perpendicular to the film
— Central ray (a) 2 FB above pelvic crest and (b) one hand's breadth
   anterior to the posterior skin border, directed to the middle of the
   cassette
— Centering and collimation, side adjacent to the film identified
— Breath held after expiration
— One view each in maximal flexion and extension

Variation
Function studies with left and right lateral bending films (film speed 400,
otherwise as for AP lumbar spine)

Tips & Tricks
If there is a marked levoscoliosis, turn left shoulder towards the cassette stand.

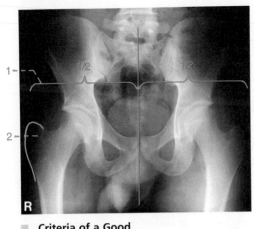

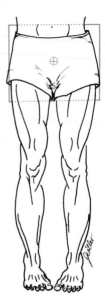

■ **Criteria of a Good Radiographic View**
— Complete and symmetrical view of the pelvis that includes hip joints, trochanters, and iliac wings (1)
— Lateral cortex of the major trochanters on both sides well delineated (2)

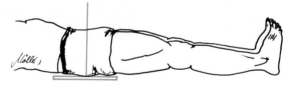

Alignment
— Projection: AP, perpendicular to the film
— Central ray directed to the middle of the cassette
— Centering, collimation, side identification
— Breath held after expiration

Imaging Technique
Film size: 14 × 17" (35 × 43 cm), crosswise
Film speed: 200 (400)
FFD: 40" (115 cm)
Bucky: yes (under the table)
Focal spot: large
Exposure: 77 kV, automatic, both outer or all three photocells

Patient Preparation
— Remove all clothes except undergarments, remove shoes

Positioning
Standing
— Patient stands with the back to the cassette stand, arms are hanging down
— Legs straight, feet slightly turned in (great toes touch, heels about 4 cm apart)
— Adjust any difference in leg length and note on the film
— Compression band across the abdomen (caution: abdominal aortic aneurysm)
Recumbent
— Supine position, legs rotated inward, both knees at the same level (if patient has difficulty straightening one knee, support the opposite side with a sponge pad)
— Upper cassette border 4 cm above pelvic crest
— Gonads shielded for males

Variations
Lower pelvic view
— Upper border of the cassette at the level of anterior superior iliac spine, otherwise as above
Pelvis, Pennal I technique
— Projection: craniocaudad 40°
— Central ray at the level of the anterior superior iliac spine, directed to the middle of the cassette
Pelvis, Pennal II technique
— Projection: caudocephalad 40°
— Central ray 4 cm below the upper border of the symphysis, directed to the middle of the cassette

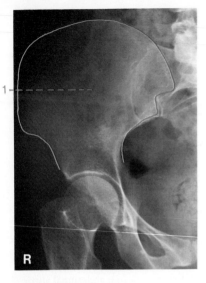

R

■ **Criteria of a Good Radiographic View**
Complete visualization of the iliac wing (1)

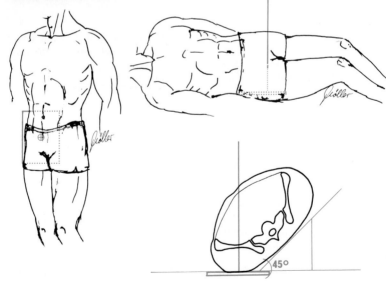

45°

Imaging Technique
Film size: 10 × 12" (24 × 30 cm), lengthwise
Film speed: 200 (400)
FFD: 40" (115 cm)
Bucky: yes (under the table)
Focal spot: large
Exposure: 77 kV, automatic, center cell

Patient Preparation
— Remove all clothes, except undergarments

Positioning

— Supine
— Elevate opposite side of the body 45° and support with sponge wedge (leave out gluteal region)
— Affected leg straight, opposite leg flexed (for support)
— Upper cassette border 2–4 cm above the pelvic crest
— Gonads shielded for males

Alignment
— Projection: oblique ventrodorsal (AP), perpendicular to the film
— Central ray directed to the middle of the cassette
— Centering, collimation, side identification

Variations
Low iliac-wing view (for anterior acetabular rim)
— As above, but central ray directed to the middle of the hip joint
Faux-profile view
— Opposite side elevated 65° instead of 45° (for a second plane of the hip joint)
— Central ray directed to the hip joint

Tips & Tricks
*A*lar = *O*ther side *a*lso (for comparison)

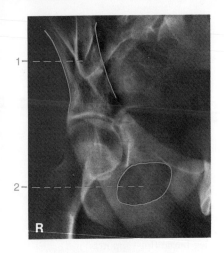

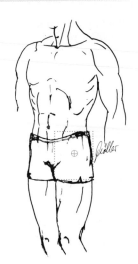

■ **Criteria of a Good Radiographic View**

— Obturator foramen horizontal–oval (2)
— Iliac wing foreshortened (1)

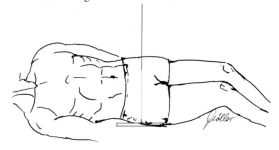

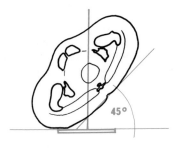

Imaging Technique

Film size: 10 × 12" (24 × 30 cm), lengthwise
Film speed: 200 (400)
FFD: 40" (115 cm)
Bucky: yes (under the table)
Focal spot: large
Exposure: 70–80 kV, automatic, center cell

Patient Preparation

— Remove all clothes, except undergarments

Positioning

— Supine
— Elevate side to be examined 45° and support with sponge wedge (under the back, leave out gluteal region)
— Affected leg straight, opposite leg flexed (for support)
— Gonads shielded for males, for females the unaffected side is shielded

Alignment

— Projection: oblique ventrodorsal (AP), perpendicular to the film
— Central ray directed to the middle of the femoral neck = midinguinal area
— Centering, collimation, side identification
— Breath held after expiration

Variation

High obturator view (at a 2nd plane of the iliac wing = alar view): central ray directed to the middle of the iliac wing, otherwise as above.

Tips & Tricks

— *Up*turator view: side to be examined *up*
— By using a larger film and centering over the midpelvis, one also gets a view of the opposite side (when looking for a fracture of the pelvic ring, for example)

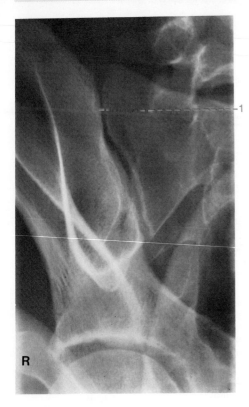

R

■ **Criteria of a Good Radiographic View**
Unobstructed projection of the sacroiliac joints (1)

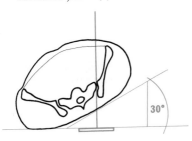

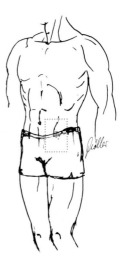

Imaging Technique
Film size: 8 × 10" (18 × 24 cm), lengthwise
Film speed: 200 (400)
FFD: 40" (115 cm)
Bucky: yes
Focal spot: large
Exposure: 77 kV, automatic, center cell

Patient Preparation
— Remove all clothes, except undergarments
— Evacuate bowel (enema if needed)

Positioning
— Supine position
— Elevate side to be examined 30°–45°
— Gonads shielded for males
— Middle of the cassette 2–3 FB below pelvic crest

Alignment
— Projection: oblique ventrodorsal (AP), perpendicular to the middle of the cassette
— Central ray 3 FB medial to the anterior superior iliac spine
— Centering, collimation, side identification
— Breath held after expiration

Tips & Tricks
Take views of both sides for comparison.

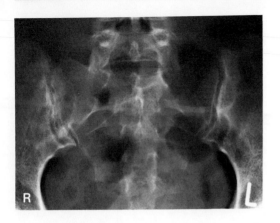

■ **Criteria of a Good Radiographic View**
Complete visualization of the sacroiliac joints

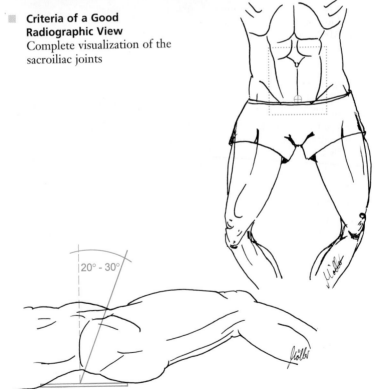

Imaging Technique

Film size: 10 × 12" 24 × 30 cm), lengthwise (or 8 × 10" [18 × 24 cm], crosswise)
Film speed: 200 (400)
FFD: 40" (115 cm)
Bucky: yes
Focal spot: large
Manual exposure: 77 kV;   …mAs,   …mAs,   …mAs

Patient Preparation

— Remove all clothes, except undergarments
— Evacuate bowel (enema if needed)

Positioning

— Supine, arms along the sides of the body
— Hips and knee joints flexed and abducted
— Gonads shielded for males
— Middle of the cassette 2–3 FB below pelvic crest

Alignment

— Projection: ventrodorsal (AP), 20°–30° caudocephalad (or vertical)
— Central ray 2 FB above the border of the symphysis
— Centering, collimation, side identification
— Breath held after expiration

Variation

Lithotomy position
— Patient draws up both legs (to reduce lordosis) and abducts the flexed legs
— Central ray vertical

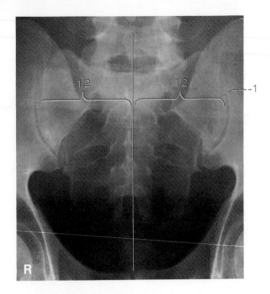

■ **Criteria of a Good Radiographic View**
Unobstructed, unforeshortened, and symmetrical (1) view of the sacrum, sacroiliac joints, and the 5th lumbar vertebra

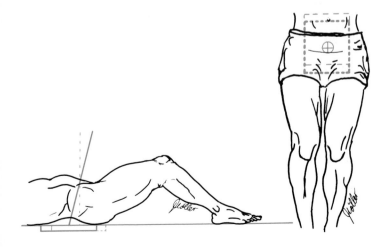

Imaging Technique
Film size: 10 × 12" (24 × 30 cm), lengthwise
Film speed: 400
FFD: 40" (115 cm)
Bucky: yes (under the table)
Focal spot: large
Exposure: 75–85 kV, automatic, center cell

Patient Preparation
— Remove all clothes, except undergarments
— Evacuate bowel (enema if needed)

Positioning

— Supine, arms along the sides of the body
— Hip and knee joints flexed (sponge support under knees)
— Gonads shielded for males
— Middle of the cassette at the level of the anterior superior iliac spine
  in median plane (lower cassette border at the level of the symphysis,
  upper cassette border at pelvic crest)

Alignment
— Projection: ventrodorsal (AP), 20° caudocephalad (or vertical)
— Central ray 2 FB above border of the symphysis (or, in vertical pro-
  jection, medial plane at the level of the anterior superior iliac
  spine), directed to the middle of the cassette
— Centering, collimation, side identification
— Breath held after expiration

Variation
Coccyx, AP projection
— Projektion: 20° craniocaudad
— Central ray a hand's breadth above the symphysis, directed to the
  middle of the cassette
— Exposure: 76 kV, automatic, center cell
— Otherwise as above

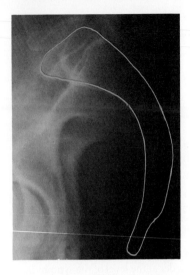

▨ Criteria of a Good Radiographic View
Lateral view shows straight and complete visualization of sacrum and coccyx

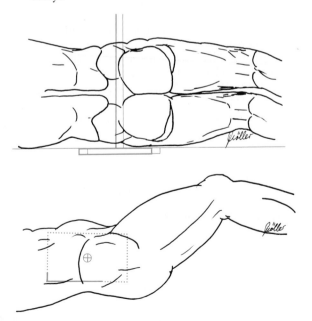

Imaging Technique
Film size: 7 × 17" (20 × 40 cm) (24 × 30 cm), lengthwise
Film speed: 400 (200–600)
FFD: 40" (115 cm)
Bucky: yes (under the table)
Focal spot: large
Exposure: 90 kV, automatic, center cell (density compensation +1)

Patient Preparation
— Remove all clothes, except undergarments

Positioning

— Straight lateral position, hips and knee joints flexed
— Sponge padding under waist and knees
— Middle of the cassette:
— Sacrum: midpoint between pelvic crest and tip of the coccyx
— Coccyx: over the lower third between pelvic crest and tip of the coccyx
— Sacrum and coccyx: a hand's breadth below the pelvic crest and a hand's breadth anterior to the posterior skin border (more anterior in obese patients)
— Gonads shielded for males

Alignment
— Projection: lateral, perpendicular to the film
— Central ray directed to the middle of the cassette (nearly one hand's breadth below the pelvic crest for the sacrum, more for the coccyx)
— Centering, collimation (identify side adjacent to the film)
— Breath held after expiration

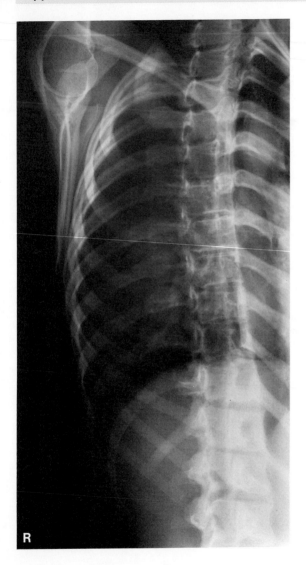

R

■ **Criteria of a Good Radiographic View**
Ribs well exposed and completely visualized

Imaging Technique

Film size: 14 × 17" (35 × 43 cm) (or 7 × 17" [20 × 40 cm] for oblique), lengthwise
Film speed: 200, compensating screen –/+
FFD: 40" (115 cm)
Bucky: yes (under the table)
Focal spot: large
Exposure: 66 kV or 73 kV (for lower ribs), automatic, center cell

Patient Preparation

— Remove all clothes from the waist up
— Remove jewelry (necklace, earrings)
— Have hair tied up on top of the head

Positioning

The injured part of the rib is always placed closest to the film:
— A. Patients stands/lies with his back (or, depending on the injury, with his chest) straight against the cassette
— Head turned to the healthy side
— Arms along the sides of the body, slightly rotated inward and abducted (hands on hips)
— Upper border of the cassette at the level the 6th cervical vertebra (above vertica prominens) (or lower border of the cassette 2 cm above pelvic crest)
— B. Healthy side turned up 30°–40°, affected side next to the film (prone or supine position)
— Gonads shielded (short lead apron)

Alignment

— Projection: perpendicular (AP or PA) to the film
— Central ray directed to the middle of the film
— Centering, collimation, side identification
— Breathing suspended after inspiration

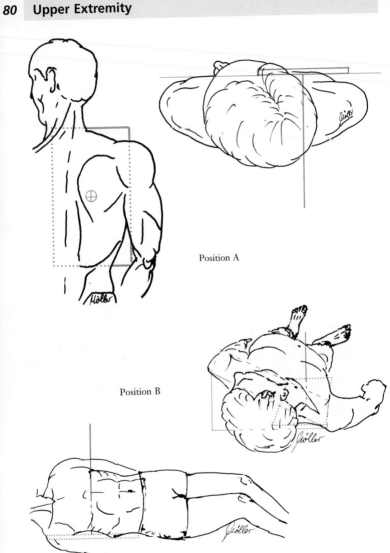

Position A

Position B

Variation

Additional views of the lower ribs:
— Film size: 10 × 12" (20 × 30 cm), lengthwise
— Supine position, healthy side elevated 45°, arms turned up
— Lower cassette border 2 FB above pelvic crest
— Breath held in expiration (diaphragms elevated: photocell over the upper abdomen = good exposure of the lower ribs)

Tips & Tricks
Mark the area that hurts.

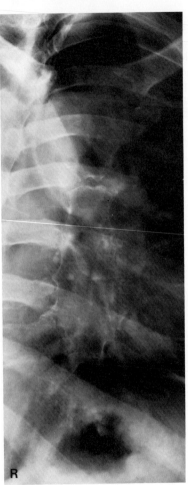

R

Criteria of a Good Radiographic View
Sternum clearly demonstrated (thoracic spine or scapula not superimposed)

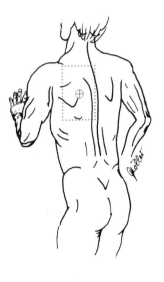

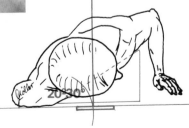

Imaging Technique

Film size: 10 × 12" (24 × 30 cm), lengtwise
Film speed: 200
FFD: 40" (115 cm)
Bucky: yes (under the table)
Focal spot: large
Exposure: 66 kV, automatic, center cell

Patient Preparation

— Remove all clothes from the waist up
— Remove jewelry (necklace, earrings)
— Have hair tied up on top of the head

Positioning

— Prone, left (right) side turned up about 20°–30°, to move sternum away from the overlying thoracic spine, and supported with the left (right) hand
— Wedge pad for additional support
— Other arm along the side of the body
— Upper cassette border 2 FB above jugular fossa
— Gonads shielded (small lead apron)

Alignment

— Projection: dorsoventral (PA), perpendicular to the film
— Central ray 3 FB left (right) of the thoracic spine (at about the level of the medial scapular border on the elevated side) directed to the middle of the film
— Centering, collimation, side identification
— Breath held after expiration

Tips & Tricks

Small patient = elevate more
Large patient = elevate less

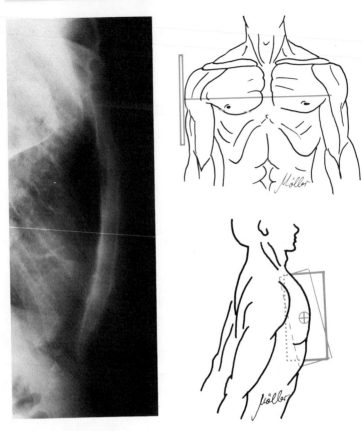

Criteria of a Good Radiographic View
Complete visualization of the sternum

Imaging Technique

Film size: 10 × 12" (24 × 30 cm) (30 × 40 cm), lengthwise
Film speed: 200
FFD: 40" (115 cm)
Bucky: yes (under the table)
Focal spot: small
Exposure: 63–77 kV, automatic, center cell

Patient Preparation

— Remove jewelry (necklace)
— Remove all clothes from the waistup

Positioning

— Patient stands with shoulder lateral to the vertical cassette stand
— Arms behind the back
— Chest pushed forward
— Upper border of the cassette 3 cm above the sternal notch
— Gonads shielded

Alignment

— Projection: lateral
— Central ray to the middle of the sternum and middle of the cassette (about 3 cm behind the anterior surface)
— Centering, collimation (place the cassette obliquely, if possible, to collimate narrowly)
— Breathing suspended in inspiration

Variation

— Lateral sternum in the recumbent position: supine, either arms extended upward or back supported with pillows with arms hanging down over the sides
— Cassettes placed upright against the side

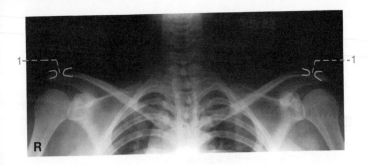

■ **Criteria of a Good Radiographic View**
Complete visualization of both acromioclavicular joints (1)

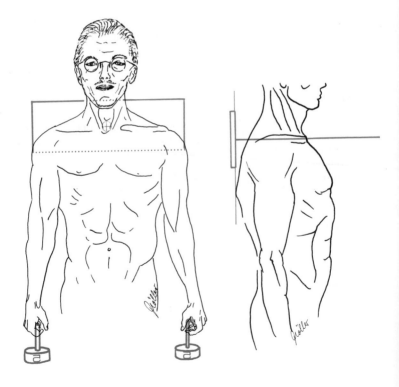

Imaging Technique

Film size: 7 × 17" (20 × 60 cm), crosswise (or larger size, collimated)
Film speed: 200
FFD: 40" (120–150 cm)
Bucky: no (tabletop exposure)
Focal spot: small
Manual exposure: 60–65 kV; 10–16 mAs, ...mAs, ...mAs, ...mAs

Patient Preparation

— Remove jewelry (necklace, earrings)
— Remove all clothes from the waist up

Positioning

— Patient with the back to the vertical cassette stand, shoulders pulled back, chest pushed out
— Arms hang along the sides of the body
— Weights (about 5–10 kg) in both hands
— Upper cassette border 2 cm above the superior margin of the shoulder
— Gonads shielded (lead apron)

Alignment

— Projection: ventrodorsal (AP), perpendicular to the film
— Central ray directed to the sternal notch and middle of the cassette; the (horizontal) transverse center passes through both acromioclavicular joints
— Centering, collimation, sides identified; "weight bearing, bilateral, 5 kg" noted on the film
— Breath held after expiration

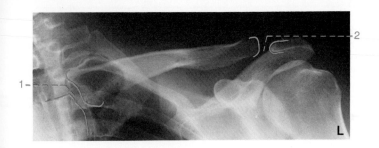

■ **Criteria of a Good Radiographic View**
Complete visualization of the clavicle, including the sternoclavicular (1) and acromioclavicular joint (2)

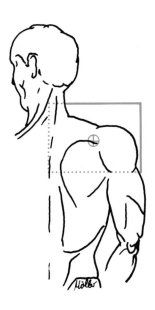

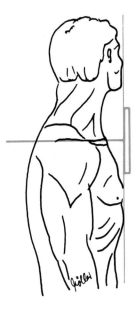

Imaging Technique

Film size: 10 × 12" (24 × 30 cm) (18 × 24 cm), crosswise
Film speed: 200
FFD: 40" (115 cm)
Bucky: yes (no)
Focal spot: small
Exposure: 66 kV, automatic, center cell (manual: 66 kV; 16–20 mAs,
…mAs,   …mAs)

Patient Preparation

— Remove jewelry (necklace, earrings)
— Remove all clothes from the waist up

Positioning

— Patient stands with the chest to the cassette stand, clavicle placed
  against the film (or supine position)
— Face turned to the opposite side
— Arm on the side to be examined rotated inward (back of the hand
  towards the stand)
— Upper cassette border 2 FB above shoulder level
— Gonads shielded (lead apron over the back)

Alignment

— Projection: dorsoventral (PA), perpendicular to the film
— Central ray directed to the midpoint of the clavicle and middle of
  the film
— Centering, collimation, side identification
— Breathing suspended in expiration

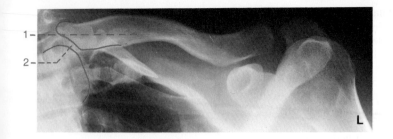

■ **Criteria of a Good Radiographic View**
— Visualization of the entire clavicle (1)
— Middle and lateral portions without superimposed shadows (with the exception of the sternoclavicular joint [2])

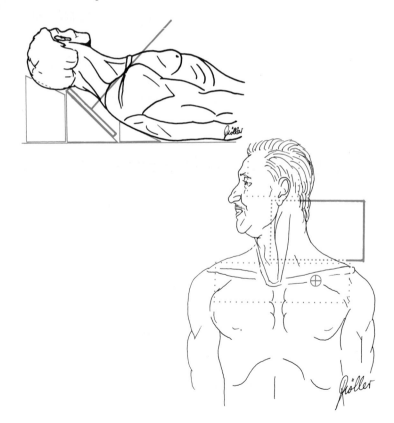

Imaging Technique
Film size: 10 × 12" (24 × 30 cm) (18 × 24 cm), crosswise
Film speed: 200
FFD: 40" (100 cm)
Bucky: no (tabletop technique)
Focal spot: small
Manual exposure: 50–66 kV; 10 mAs,   …mAs,   …mAs

Patient Preparation
— Remove jewelry (necklace, earrings)
— Remove all clothes from the waist up

Positioning

— Supine position, arms along the sides of the body, head turned to the opposite side
— Shoulder and head slightly elevated and supported with sponge pad
— Cassette placed against the back of the shoulder at an oblique angle of about 45° to the tabletop (and supported with a wedge, additional sandbag if needed)
— Gonads shielded (lead apron)

Alignment
— Projection: 45° cephalad angulation (oblique ventrocaudad to dorsocephalad [oblique AP]) perpendicular to the film
— Central ray directed to the midpoint of the clavicle and middle of the film
— Centering, collimation, side identification
— Breath held after expiration

Variation
— Patient in supine position (or stands with the back to the vertical grid)
— Healthy shoulder slightly elevated (supported) until clavicle is parallel to the cassette
— Hand on the side to be examined is supinated
— Projection: 30° caudocephalad
— Central ray directed to the midpoint of the clavicle and the middle of the film
— Exposure: 55 kV, automatic, center cell

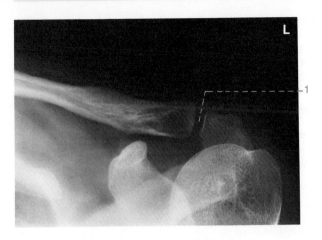

■ **Criteria of a Good Radiographic View**
Unobstructed view of the acromioclavicular joint (1)

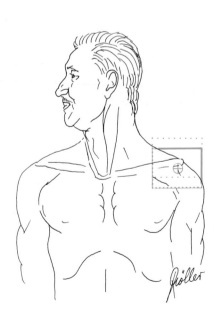

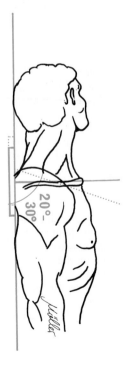

Imaging Technique
Film size: 8 × 10" (18 × 24 cm) (13 × 18 cm), crosswise
Film speed: 200
FFD: 40" (100 cm)
Bucky: yes (no), under the table (tabletop)
Focal spot: small
Exposure: 57–60 kV, automatic, center cell (manual: 57–60 kV, 10 mAs, …mAs, ….mAs)

Patient Preparation
— Remove jewelry (necklace)
— Remove all clothes from the waist up

Positioning

— Patient sitting or lying with the back to the film
— Arms along the sides of the body, inside of the hand turned out
— Upper cassette border 2 cm above the superior margin of the shoulder in vertical projection, higher if the tube is angled
— Gonads shielded (lead apron)

Alignment
— Projection: ventrodorsal (AP), perpendicular to the film (perhaps 20°–35° caudocephalad)
— Central ray directed to the acromioclavicular joint
— Centering, collimation, side identification
— Breath held after expiration

Tips & Tricks
— This view is also taken as a 3rd view of the shoulder joint (see p. 99)
— A compensating filter may be used if available

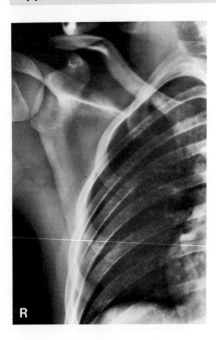

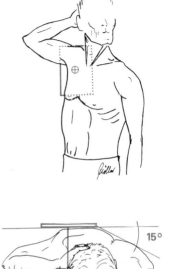

Position A

■ **Criteria of a Good Radiographic View**
Complete visualization of the scapula, no ribs overlying the lateral portion

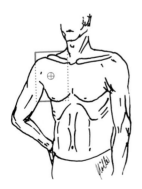

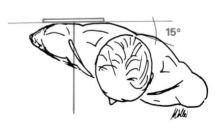

Position B

Imaging Technique
Film size: 10 × 12" (24 × 30 cm), lengthwise
Film speed: 200
FFD: 40" (115 cm)
Bucky: yes (vertical bucky grid)
Focal spot: small
Exposure: 66 kV, automatic, center cell

Patient Preparation
— Remove jewelry (necklace, earrings)
— Remove all clothes from the waist up

Positioning

— Patient with the back and scapula flat against the upright cassette stand
— The unaffected side is elevated 15° (scapula parallel to the film)
— Chin lifted, head turned to the opposite side
— Hand on the affected side turned up and put on top of the head (A), or placed on the hip (arm abducted, B)
— Upper cassette border at the level of the superior border of the shoulder
— Gonads shielded (small lead apron)

Alignment
— Projection: ventrodorsal (AP), perpendicular to the film
— Central ray directed to the midpoint of the scapula and middle of the film
— Centering, collimation, side identification
— Breathing suspended in expiration

Tips & Tricks
The middle of the scapula lies 4 FB below the clavicle and 1 FB lateral to the mamillary line.

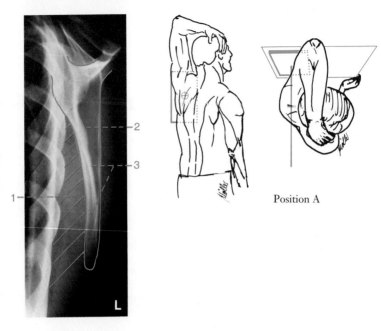

Position A

■ **Criteria of a Good Radiographic View**
— Clear space between ribs and scapula (1)
— Complete demonstration of the entire scapula (2)
— Lateral and medial border of the scapula superimposed (3)

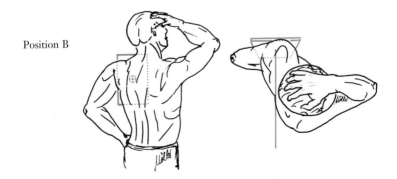

Position B

Imaging Technique

Film size: 10 × 12" (24 × 30 cm), lengthwise
Film speed: 200
FFD: 40" (115 cm)
Bucky: yes (under the table)
Focal spot: small
Exposure: 66 kV, automatic, center cell

Patient Preparation

— Remove jewelry (necklace, earrings)
— Remove all clothes from the waist up

Positioning

— Patient with the appropriate shoulder lateral to the upright cassette
  stand
— Hand on that side placed on top of the head (A) or resting on the
  hip (B) (arm abducted); the other shoulder turned slightly forward
  (arm of the unaffected side held in front), so that medial and lateral
  borders of the scapula to be examined are superimposed (check by
  palpating between thumb and forefinger!)
— Lower cassette border 2–5 cm below the inferior angle of the
  scapula
— Gonads shielded (small lead apron, on the side)

Alignment

— Projection: tangential to the scapula (slightly oblique lateral, per-
  pendicular to the film)
— Central ray directed to the midpoint of the scapula (about middle of
  the axilla) and middle of the film
— Centering, collimation, side identification
— Breathing suspended

Variation

Scapula, oblique projection, Neer and Larché technique (for injured
patients)
— Supine position (or back to the upright stand), affected side elevated
  45°, upper arm along the side, forearm flexed, resting on the abdomen
— Projection: ventrodorsal (AP) oblique, perpendicular to the cassette
— Central ray directed through the upper arm and the space between ribs
  and scapula at the level of the axillary fold, to the middle of the cassette

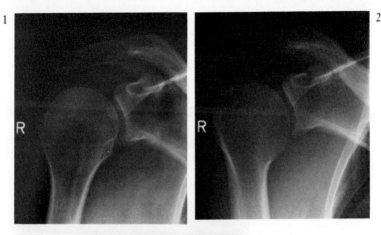

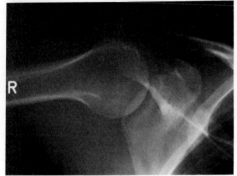

■ **Criteria of a Good Radiographic View**
Complete and unobstructed visualization
of the head of the humerus and of the
shoulder joint

Imaging Technique
Film size: 8 × 10" (18 × 24 cm), crosswise (or 10 × 12", lengthwise)
Film speed: 200
FFD: 40" (115 cm)
Bucky: yes (under the table)
Focal spot: small
Exposure: 65–70 kV, automatic, center cell

Patient Preparation
— Remove jewelry (necklace, earrings)
— Remove all clothes from the waist up

Positioning

Positions 1 and 2
— Patient stands with the scapula flat against the vertical cassette stand, the opposite side of the back is turned 45° away from the stand
— The arm on the affected side is placed adjacent to the cassette, the elbow is flexed 90°, the hand is supinated, palm of the hand turned up
— Internal rotation (1): forearm is placed on the abdomen
— External rotation (2): forearm is turned out (and may hold on to the cassette stand)
Position 3
— Abduction (3): back flat against the cassette stand (straight, not rotated), arm abducted at a right angle, forearm flexed 90° and extended upward, palm of the hand turned forward (may hold on to an i.v. pole, for instance)
— Upper cassette border 2 cm above the superior margin of the shoulder
— Compensating filter for positions 1 and 2
— Gonads shielded (lead apron)

Alignment
— Projection: for 1 and 2: oblique ventrodorsal (AP), 15°–20° craniocaudad
— For 3; ventrodorsal, perpendicular to the middle of the cassette
— Central ray for 1 and 2 directed to the center of the head of the humerus and middle of the film; for 3, perpendicular to the joint space
— Centering, collimation, side identification
— Breathing suspended in expiration

Projection for
Positions 1 and 2
(for position 3 =
vertical = dotted line)

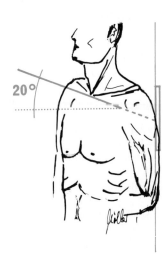

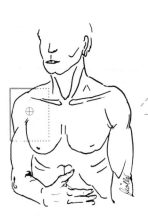

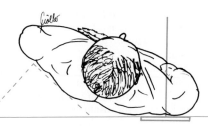

Position 1

Tips & Tricks
— Center of the humeral head = 3 FB below the clavicle
— Use an i.v. pole for something to grasp and hold onto

Position 2

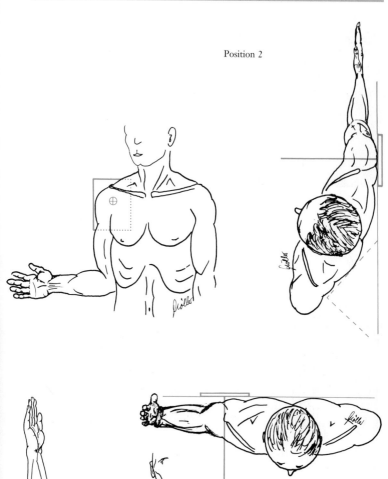

Position 3

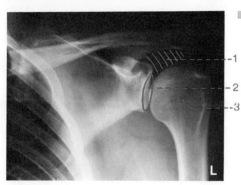

■ **Criteria of a Good Radiographic View**

— Complete, unobstructed view of the humeral head and shoulder joint (3)
— Glenoid fossa linear or small oval (2)
— Clear view of the subacromial space (1)

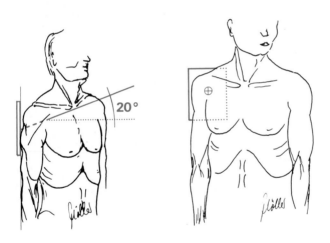

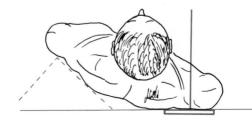

Imaging Technique
Film size: 8 × 10" (18 × 24 cm), lengthwise   Film speed: 200
FFD: 40" (115 cm)   Bucky: yes (under the table)   Focal spot: small
Exposure: 60–66 kV, automatic, center cell

Patient Preparation
— Remove all clothes from the waist up and all jewelry

Positioning

— Scapula adjacent to and parallel to the cassette, opposite side rotated about 45° away from the upright stand (use sponge wedge for support)
— Arm along the side of the body, hanging down, hand supinated
— Head turned the other way (for radiation protection)
— Upper cassette border 2 cm above the superior margin of the shoulder
— Shoulder filter, if needed
— Gonads shielded (lead apron)

Alignment
— Projection: oblique ventrodorsal (AP) (perhaps 20° craniocaudad, although not in cases of possible fracture or dislocation)
— Central ray perpendicular to the joint space, and directed to the middle of the film
— Centering, collimation, side identification
— Breath held after expiration

Variation
Shoulder in 2 planes
— Extend the arm straight upward (above the head), otherwise as above (shoulder, axial projection, see p. 105)
Glenohumeral joint, profile view, Bernageau position
— Shoulder to be examined turned to the stand
— Arm in maximal abduction, forearm extended above the head, opposite side rotated about 20°–30° anteriorly
— Projection: lateral, 25°–30° craniocaudad
— Central ray 2 cm below the skin fold or the top of the acromion and 2 cm towards the spine, directed to the middle of the cassette
Grashey position (lateral process of the scapula)
— Affected arm in internal rotation, projection perpendicular to the film, otherwise as above

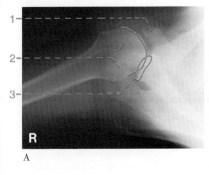

A

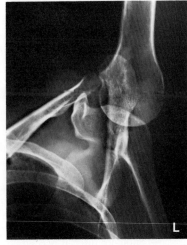

C

■ **Criteria of a Good Radiographic View**
— Joint surfaces (outlined) and joint space well demonstrated
— Unobstructed view of the coracoid process (1)
— Acromioclavicular joint projected over the humerus (2)
— Inferior glenoid rim clearly demonstrated (3)

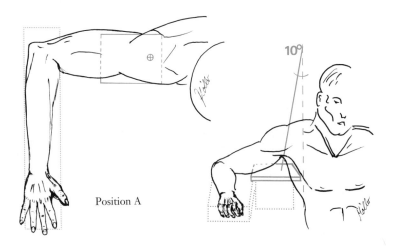

Position A

10°

Imaging Technique
Film size: 8 × 10" (18 × 24 cm), lengthwise
Film speed: 200
FFD: 40" (100 cm)
Bucky: no (tabletop technique)
Focal spot: small
Exposure: 65–70 kV;   …mAs,   …mAs,   …mAs
or (for position C) automatic, center cell

Patient Preparation
— Remove jewelry (necklace, earrings)
— Remove all clothes from the waist up

Positioning

— A. Patient sits at the side of the table; the arm is abducted about
    45°, elbow flexed 90°, forearm lies on the table (cassette may be
    supported), forearm pronated and parallel to the plane of the
    table
— B. Patient supine, shoulder and upper arm supported, upper arm
    abducted 90°, forearm supinated (palm of the hand turned up),
    elevated on wooden board
    Cassette placed in vertical position, cephalad, on the radial side
    of the shoulder, and supported with sandbags
    Patient's head inclined all the way to the opposite side
— C. Patient with the back to the stand, arm on the affected side
    raised vertically, forearm flexed 90° at the elbow and placed on
    top of the head
    Patient's head inclined to the opposite side
— Gonads shielded (lead apron)

Alignment
— Projection:
    A. Oblique, 5°–10°, from cranial–medial to caudal–lateral
    B. Oblique, 5°–10°, from caudal–lateral to cranial–medial
    C. Vertical ventrodorsal (AP)
— Central ray directed to the center of the joint space and middle of
  the film
— Centering, collimation, side identification
— Breath held after expiration

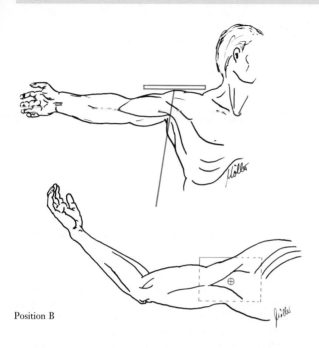

Position B

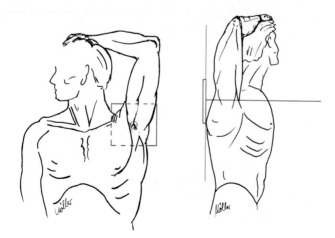

Position C

Imaging Technique
Film size: 8 × 10" (18 × 24 cm), crosswise
Film speed: 200
FFD: 40" (100 cm)
Bucky: no (tabletop technique)
Focal spot: small
Manual exposure: 50–55 kV; 10 mAs,   …mAs,   …mAs

Patient Preparation
— Remove jewelry (necklace, earrins)
— Remove all clothes from the waist up

Positioning

Hermodsson position
— Supine, hand of the side being examined resting on the opposite shoulder
— Cassette perpendicular to the table behind the shoulder, parallel to the clavicle (lateral side of the cassette moved about 20° toward the head)
Johner position
— Supine, upper arm of the side being examined along the side, forearm flexed 90°, resting on the abdomen
— Cassette on the table behind the shoulder, perpendicular to the central ray
— Have patient turn the head to the other side (radiation protection)
— Gonads shielded (large lead apron)

Alignment
1 (Hermodsson)
— Projection: parallel to the table, 20° lateromedial
— Central ray perpendicular to the cassette, directed to the midpoint of the humeral head and the middle of the cassette
2 (Johner)
— Projection: oblique horizontal, 20° from lateral to medial, and 20° from caudal to cranial, to the axis of the upper arm of the same side (from laterodorsal to mediocranial)
— Central ray perpendicular to the middle of the cassette
— Centering, collimation, side identification
— Breath held after expiration

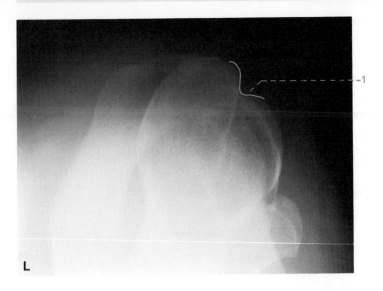

L

■ **Criteria of a Good Radiographic View**
Bicipital groove free of superimposed shadows (1)

Variations

West-Point View

— Prone, upper part of the body on broad sponge pad, the arm being examined hangin straight down
— Cassette perpendicular to the table, upright on edge behind the shoulder
— Projection: inferior oblique, 25° from posterior to anterior, and 25° from lateral to medial
— Central ray directed to the joint space and middle of the cassette

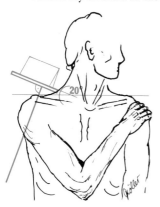

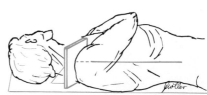

Position 1 (Hermodsson)

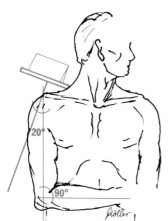

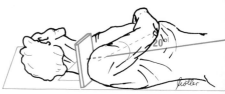

Position 2 (Johner)

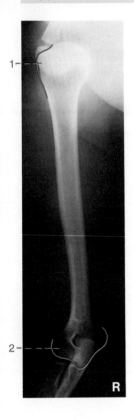

▓ **Criteria of a Good Radiographic View**

— Complete visualization of the entire humerus, including both joints if possible

— AP projection of the trochlea of the humerus (2)

— The greater tubercle presents as the lateral border (1)

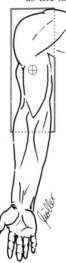

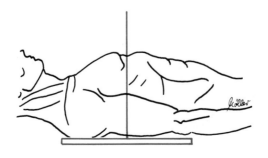

Imaging Technique

Film size: 7 × 17" (18 × 43 cm) (20 × 40 cm), lengthwise
Film speed: 200, compensating screen +/–
FFD: 40" (115 cm)
Bucky: yes/no (under the table/tabletop technique)
Focal spot: small
Exposure: 60–66 kV, automatic, center cell (or manual: 60 kV;
20 mAs,   …mAs,   …mAs)

Patient Preparation

— Remove jewelry (necklace, earrings)
— Remove all clothes from the waist up

Positioning

— Patient with the back to the stand (on the bucky table)
— Back of the upper arm placed against the cassette (unaffected side slightly rotated forward or elevated)
— Arm somewhat abducted but in contact with the film
— Hand supinated (palm forward = external rotation)
— Upper cassette border 2 cm above the superior border of the shoulder
— Head turned to the opposite side
— Gonads shielded (lead apron)

Alignment

— Projection: ventrodorsal, perpendicular to the film
— Central ray directed to the midpoint of the upper arm and middle of the cassette
— Centering, collimation, side identification
— Breathing suspended

Tips & Tricks

If external rotation is too painful, turn the entire body with the healthy side forward (or elevate the side) to bring the upper arm adjacent to the film

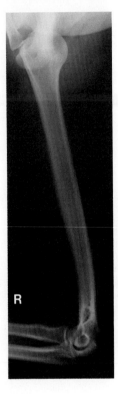

Criteria of a Good Radiographic View

Complete visualization of the entire humerus, including at least one joint (both joints if possible), elbow joint in straight lateral projection

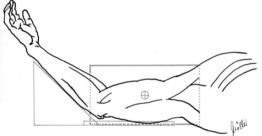

Position A

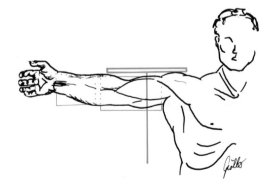

Imaging Technique
Film size: 7 × 17" (18 × 43 cm), lengthwise
Film speed: 200 or 100, compensating screen +/–
FFD: 40" (100 cm)
Bucky: yes (no)
Focal spot: small
Exposure: 66 kV, automatic, center cell (manual: 66 kV;
20 mAs,   …mAs,   …mAs)

Patient Preparation
— Remove jewelry (necklace, earrings)
— Remove all clothes from the waist up

Positioning

— A. Patient supine, upper arm abducted 90°, forearm supinated (elevated and supported on a wooden board), palm of the hand turned up. Cassette placed on edge against the radial side of the upper arm (from cephalad, so to speak), vertical, and supported with sandbags
— B. Patient sits at the side of the table, upper arm abducted 90°, elbow flexed 90°, forearm rests on the table in the same plane as the upper arm (support if necessary), hand extended straight
— C. Patient with the back to the stand (unaffected side slightly raised), upper arm abducted 90° and rotated externally (forearm elevated, elbow flexed 90°, back of the forearm adjacent to the upright stand)
— Head turned to the opposite side
— Gonads shielded (large lead apron)

Alignment
— Projection: lateral (mediodorsal), perpendicular to the film (projection A from the front, B from below, C from above)
— Central ray to midhumerus and middle of the film
— Centering, collimation, side identification
— Breath held after expiration

Position B

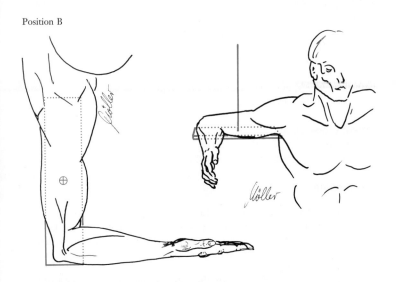

Position C

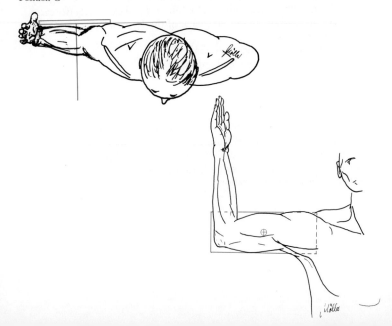

Variation

If the patient is unable to abduct the upper arm:

— Patient supine, upper portion of the body elevated (on a long sponge pad), arm along the side of the body, hand supinated
— Cassette on edge, upright between the chest wall and the inside of the upper arm, pushed as far into the axilla as possible
— Lateral projection, otherwise as above

Tips & Tricks

— Use i.v. pole for the hand to hold onto
— If there is no compensating screen available, use a bag with rice flour or a wedge filter

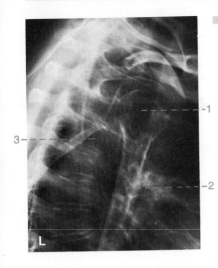

Criteria of a Good Radiographic View

Projection of the humeral head (1) and humerus (2) between the dorsal spine (3) and the sternum (by slightly rotating the unaffected side posteriorly)

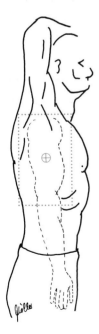

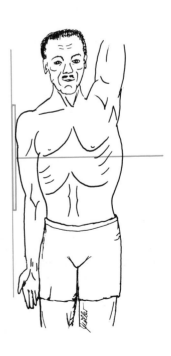

Imaging Technique

Film size: 10 × 12" (24 × 30 cm), lengthwise
Film speed: 200
FFD: 40" (115 cm)
Bucky: yes (under the table)
Focal spot: large
Exposure: 83 kV, automatic, center cell

Patient Preparation

— Remove jewelry (necklace, earrings)
— Remove all clothes from the waist up

Positioning

— Patient stands sideways, with the affected shoulder turned to the stand
— Arm on that side hanging down, hand supinated
— Opposite arm extended above the head
— Unaffected shoulder rotated slightly back
— Upper cassette border 2 cm above the superior border of the shoulder
— Gonads shielded (small lead apron)

Alignment

— Projection: lateral, perpendicular to the film
— Central ray directed to the humeral head being examined (midpoint between the axilla and the nipple of the unaffected side) and middle of the cassette
— Centering, collimation, side identification
— Breathing suspended

Tips & Tricks

Use the vertigraph for centering by positioning the center photocell over the head of the humerus, then aligning the X-ray tube with the center of the vertigraph.

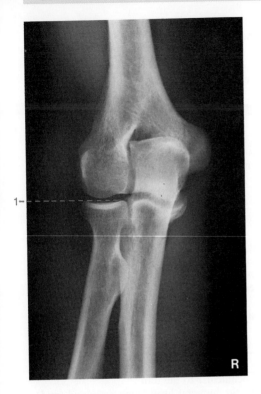

■ **Criteria of a Good Radiographic View**
Joint space in the center of the film and clearly
demonstrated (1)

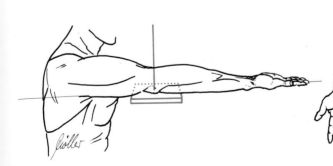

Imaging Technique

Film size: 8 × 10" (18 × 24 or 24 × 30 cm), crosswise (divided, one-half covered)
Film speed: 100
FFD: 40" (100 cm)
Bucky: no
Focal spot: small
Manual exposure: 50–55 kV; 16–20 mAs;   …mAs,   …mAs

Patient Preparation
— Remove everything from the arm

Positioning

— Patient sits at the side of the table, (legs *not* unter the table)
— Elbow joint extended, rests with the posterior (dorsal) surface on the cassette, palm turned up (supinated)
— Shoulder, elbow joint, and wrist joint in the same plane, either elevated (sponge or box), or patient's adjustable stool lowered
— Gonads shielded (large lead apron)

Alignment
— Projection: ventro-(volo-)dorsal, perpendicular to the film
— Central ray directed to the middle of the elbow joint and of the cassette
— Centering, collimation, side identififcation

Tips & Tricks
— Put a sandbag on the wrist
— If patient cannot fully extend the elbow, two exposures should be made: one each of the upper arm and of the forearm, each placed on the film

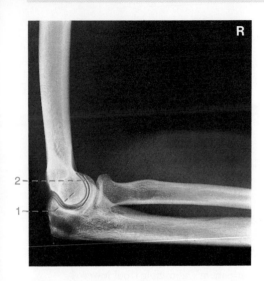

■ **Criteria of a Good Radiographic View**
— True lateral projection
— Humeroulnar joint space sharply outlined (2)
— Humeral condyles superimposed (1)

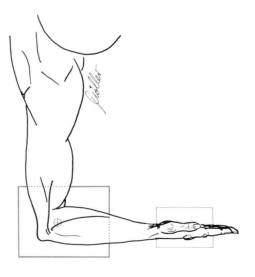

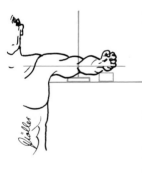

Imaging Technique
Film size: 8 × 10" (18 × 24 or 24 × 30 cm), crosswise (divided, one-half covered)
Film speed: 100
FFD: 40" (105 cm)
Bucky: no
Focal spot: small
Manual exposure: 50–55 kV; 16–20 mAs;   ...mAs,   ...mAs

Patient Prepration
— Remove everything from the arm

Positioning

— Patient sits at the side of the table, (legs *not* under the table)
— Upper arm and forearm in the same plane (either supported on box or stool lowered)
— Elbow joint flexed 90°, rests with the inside (inferior border) on the cassette
— Wrist in lateral position (thumb up)
— Gonads shielded (large lead apron)

Alignment
— Projection: lateral radioulnar, perpendicular to film
— Central ray directed to the midpoint of the elbow joint, near the center of the film
— Centering, collimation, side identification

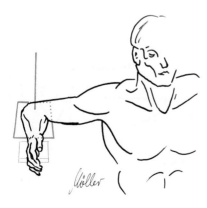

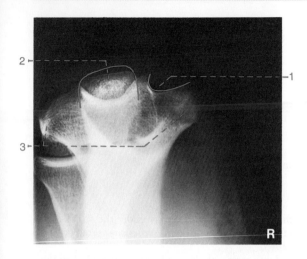

■ **Criteria of a Good Radiographic View**
— Tangential projection of the ulnar sulcus (1)
— Olecranon (2), trochlea, and the epicondyles (3) are well visualized
— Arm and forearm are superimposed

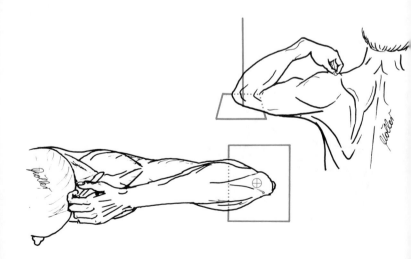

Imaging Technique
Film size: 8 × 10" (13 × 18 cm lengthwise or 18 × 24 cm crosswise)
Film speed: 100
FFD: 40" (105 cm)
Bucky: no
Focal spot: small
Manual exposure: 50 kV; 12–16 mAs,   …mAs,   …mAs

Patient Preparation
— Remove everything from the arm

Positioning

— Patient sits at the side of the table
— Arm abducted at a right angle
— Distal portion of the upper arm rests on the cassette
— Elbow joint in maximal flexion (inside of the hand on the shoulder)
— Gonads shielded (large lead apron)

Alignment
— Projection: perpendicular (ulnohumeral) to the olecranon and to
   the film
— Central ray directed to the elbow joint (about 2–3 cm below the
   olecranon) and to the middle of the film
— Centering, collimation, side identification

Variation
— Patient sits with the back to the table
— Forearm is placed on the cassette, the upper arm is at a 25°–30° angle
   to the vertical plane
— Projection humeroulnar (otherwise as above)

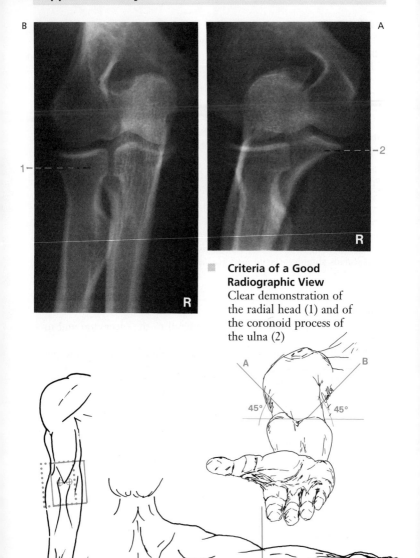

■ **Criteria of a Good Radiographic View**
Clear demonstration of the radial head (1) and of the coronoid process of the ulna (2)

Imaging Technique

Film size: 8 × 10" (18 × 24 cm), lengthwise
Film speed: 100
FFD: 40" (100 cm)
Bucky: no
Focal spot: small
Manual exposure: 50–55 kV; 16–20 mAs,   …mAs,   ….mAs

Patient Preparation

— Remove everything from the arm

Positioning

— Patient sits at the side of the table, (legs *not* under the table)
— The extended elbow joint rests with the posterior (dorsal) surface on the cassette, palm turned up (supinated)
— Shoulder, elbow joint, and wrist joint in the same plane, either elevated (sponge or box) or patient's adjustable stool lowered
— Gonads shielded (large lead apron)

Alignment

Radial head (B)
— Projection: oblique, 45° ulnoradial (medioventral–laterodorsal)
— Central ray directed to the middle of the elbow joint, 1 cm to the ulnar side (toward little finger), and middle of the film
Coronoid process of the ulna (A)
— Projection: oblique, 45° radioulnar (lateroventral–mediodorsal)
— Central ray directed to the middle of the elbow joint, 1 cm to the radial side (toward the thumb)
— Collimate closely to the size of the part and identify the sides

Tips & Tricks

— Midpoint of the elbow joint: transverse centering about 1 FB below the medial epicondyle of the humerus
— Place a sandbag on the wrist

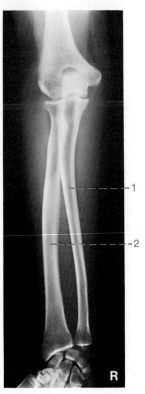

—1

—2

R

Criteria of a Good Radiographic View
Ulna (1) and radius (2) visualized in their entire length, without being superimposed, and with at least one joint demonstrated (A = with the wrist joint, B = with the elbow joint)

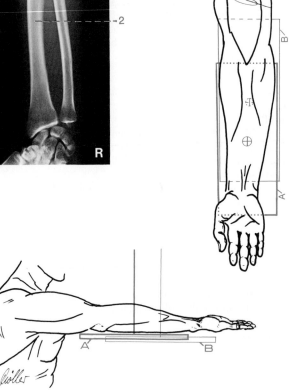

Imaging Technique
Film size: 10 × 12" (24 × 30 cm), lengthwise: (divided; one-half covered with a lead mask)
Film speed: 100
FFD: 40" (105 cm)
Bucky: no
Focal spot: small
Manual exposure: 50 kV, 16 mAs,   …mAs,   …mAs

Patient Preparation
— Remove everything from the arm
— Remove jewelry

Positioning

— Patient sits at the side of the table, (legs *not* under the table)
— The extended forearm rests with the posterior (dorsal) surface on the cassette
— Palm turned up (supinated)
— Shoulder, elbow joint, and wrist joint in the same plane, either elevated (sponge) or patient's adjustable stool lowered
— Gonads shielded (large lead apron)

Alignment
— Projection: ventro-(volo-)dorsal, perpendicular to the film
— Central ray directed to the middle of the forearm and of the film
— Centering, collimation, side identification

Tips & Tricks
— Immobilize the fingers with a sandbag
— Use a bag with rice flour to compensate for density differences

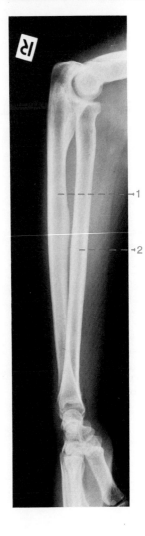

■ **Criteria of a Good Radiographic View**
— Ulna (1) and radius (2) straight lateral (their distal third superimposed)
— Wrist and elbow joint in straight lateral projection

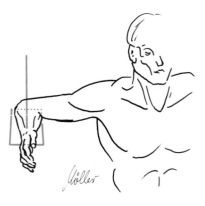

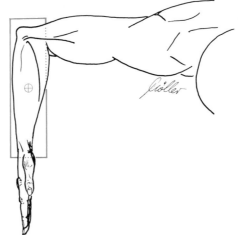

Imaging Technique

Film size: 10 × 12" (24 × 30 cm), lengthwise (divided; one-half covered with a lead mask)
Fillm speed: 100
FFD: 40" (100 cm)
Bucky: no (tabletop technique)
Focal spot: small
Manual exposure: 50–55 kV; 16 mAs,   …mAs,   …mAs

Patient Preparation
— Remove everything from the arm
— Remove jewelry

Positioning

— Patient sits at the side of the table (legs *not* under the table)
— Arm elevated and abducted, the elbow flexed 90°
— Forearm rests with the ulnar side on the cassette, straight lateral (wrist joint lateral, little finger down, thumb and fingers extended)
— Midforearm centered over the middle of the film
— Gonads shielded (large lead apron)

Alignment
— Projection: lateral radioulnar, perpendicular to the film
— Central ray directed to the middle of the forearm and middle of the film
— Centering, collimation, side identification

Tips & Tricks
— Rest the fingers against a right-angle sponge wedge
— Use a bag with rice flour to compensate for density differences

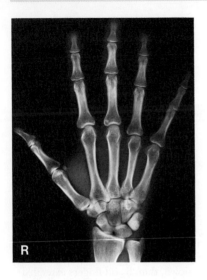

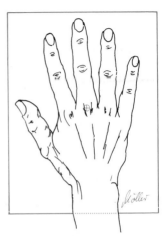

■ **Criteria of a Good Radiographic View**
Entire hand visualized, including fingertips and wrist joint

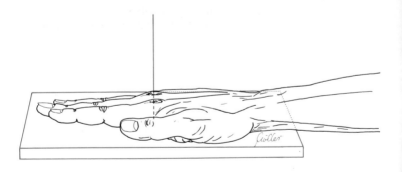

Imaging Technique
Film size: 10 × 12" (24 × 30 cm), crosswise (divided; one-half covered with a lead mask)
Film speed: 100
FFD: 40" (100 cm)
Bucky: no (tabletop exposure)
Focal spot: small
Manual exposure: 48–50 kV; 8–10 mAs,   …mAs,   …mAs

Patient Preparation
— Remove everything from the forearm
— Remove jewelry (ring, watch)

Positioning

— Patient sits at the side of the table (legs *not* under the table)
— Forearm rests on the table
— Palm of the hand rests flat on the cassette, fingers slightly spread
— Metacarpophalangeal joint of the middle finger in the center of the film
— Gonads shielded (lead apron)

Alignment
— Projection: dorsovolar (PA), perpendicular to the film
— Central ray directed to the MP joint of the middle finger and middle of the film
— Centering, collimation, side identification

Tips & Tricks
Place a sandbag across the proximal forearm.

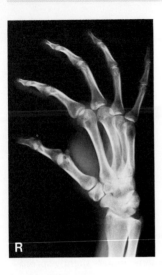

■ **Criteria of a Good Radiographic View**
Hand completely visualized, including fingertips and wrist joint

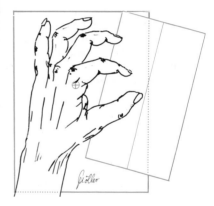

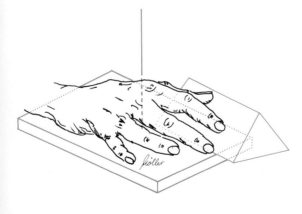

Imaging Technique

Film size: 10 × 12" (24 × 30 cm), crosswise (divided; one-half covered with a lead mask)
Film speed: 100
FFD: 40" (105 cm)
Bucky: no
Focal spot: small
Manual exposure: 46–50 kV; 10 mAs,　　…mAs,　　…mAs

Patient Preparation

— Remove everything from the forearm
— Remove jewelry (ring watch)

Positioning

— Patient sits at the side of the table (legs *not* under the table)
— Forearm rests on the table in pronation (palm down)
— Radial aspect of the hand slightly raised (thumb and index finger supported on a sponge wedge)
— Fingers spread and slightly flexed (fanned)
— Metacarpophalangeal joint of the index finger in the center of the film
— Gonads shielded (large lead apron)

Alignment

— Projection: dorsovolar, perpendicular to the film
— Central ray directed to the MP joint of the index finger in the middle of the film
— Centering, collimation, side identification

Variation

Norgaad position
— Back of the hand rests on the film, thumbside raised about 30° (sponge wedge)
— Fingers slightly bent (ballplayer view)

Tips & Tricks

Place a sandbag across the proximal forearm.

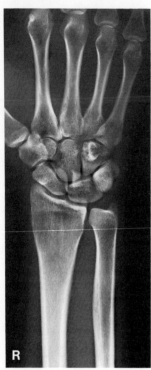

R

▓ **Criteria of a Good Radiographic View**
Wrist joint visualized completely (metacarpals, carpal bones, distal forearm)

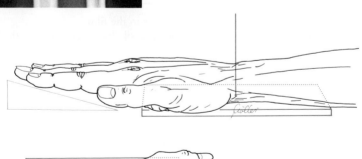

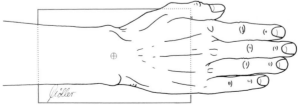

Imaging Technique
Film size: 8 × 10" (18 × 24 or 13 × 18 cm), crosswise (divided; one-half covered with lead mask)
Film speed: 100
FFD: 40" (105 cm)
Bucky: no
Focal spot: small
Manual exposure: 44–50 kV, 16–20 mAs,   …mAs,   …mAs

Patient Preparation
— Remove everything from the forearm
— Remove jewelry (ring, watch)

Positioning

— Patient sits at the side of the table (legs *not* under the table)
— Forearm and hand resting on the table in a straight line
— Volar surface of the wrist joint extended and level, resting on the center of the cassette: put a flat sponge pad under the fingers, or have the patient make a flat fist
— Gonads shielded (lead apron)

Alignment
— Projection: dorsovolar (PA), perpendicular to the film
— Central ray directed to the center of the wrist joint and middle of the film
— Centering, collimation, side identification

Tips & Tricks
— Put a sandbag across the proximal forearm
— For taking films through a cast (and in children), use film speed 200

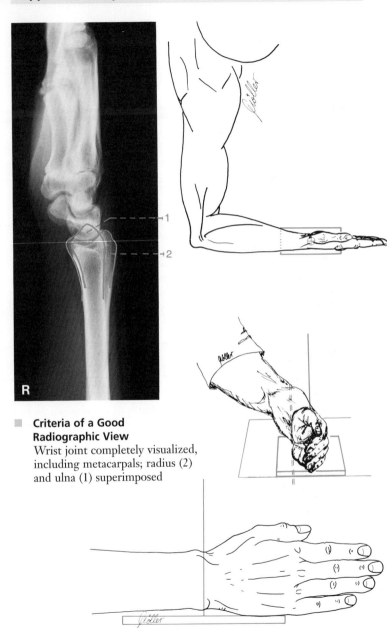

■ **Criteria of a Good Radiographic View**
Wrist joint completely visualized, including metacarpals; radius (2) and ulna (1) superimposed

Imaging Technique

Film size: 8 × 10" (18 × 24 cm), lengthwise (divided; one-half covered with lead mask

Film speed: 100

FFD: 40" (100 cm)

Bucky: no (tabletop technique)

Focal spot: small

Manual exposure: 48 kV; 20 mAs, ...mAs, ...mAs
52 kV; 64 mAs, ...mAs, ...mAs

Patient Preparation

— Remove everything from the forearm

— Remove jewelry (ring, watch)

Positioning

— Patient sits at the side of the table (legs *not* under the table)

— Wrist straight lateral, ulnar (little finger) side rests on the cassette (forearm and hand in one line)

— Thumb on the opposed side, not abducted

— Gonads shielded (large lead apron)

Alignment

— Projection: lateral (radioulnar), perpendicular to the film

— Central ray directed to the center of the wrist and middle of the film

— Centering, collimation, side identification

Tips & Tricks

— Place a sandbag across the forearm

— Turn the hand so that thenar eminence (thumb) and hypothenar eminence (little finger) are superimposed

— Patient bends over to the "healthy side" = this facilitates the superimposition of radius and ulna

— Place the hand against a 90° sponge wedge

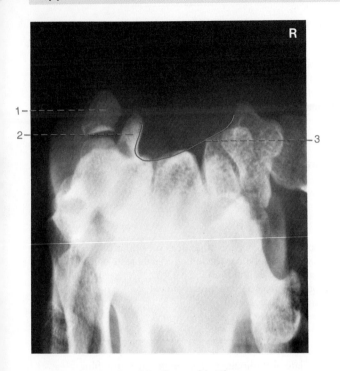

■ **Criteria of a Good Radiographic View**
Pisiform bone (1), the hamular process of the hamate (2) and the carpal tunnel (3) are clearly demonstrated

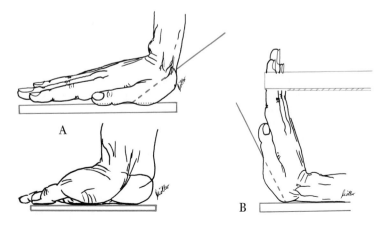

Imaging Technique

Film size: 8 × 10" (13 × 18 cm or 18 × 24 cm), lengthwise
Film speed: 100
FFD: 40" (100 cm)
Bucky: no (tabletop technique)
Focal spot: small
Manual exposure: 48 kV; 25 mAs,   …mAs,   …mAs

Patient Preparation

— Remove everything from the forearm
— Remove jewelry (ring, watch)

Positioning

— A. The standing patient puts hand on the cassette in maximal dor-
    siflexion, palmar surface down
— B. Patient sits at the side of the table (legs *not* under the table)
— Palm of the hand and distal forearm rest on the cassette
— The hand is lifted up and hyperextended in maximal dorsiflexion
    with the opposite hand (or a band)
— Wrist in the center of the film
— Gonads shielded (large lead apron)

Alignment

— Projection: oblique, 40°–45°
— Central ray directed tangentially to the carpal tunnel to the mid-
    point of the film
— Centering, collimation, side identification

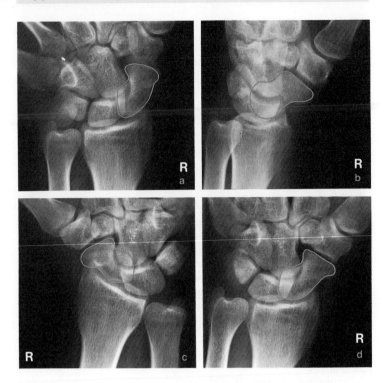

■ **Criteria of a Good Radiographic View**
   — Complete visualization of the navicular bone (outlined) in different projections
   — Navicular bone IV (variation): radius and ulna as well as the navicular and lunate are superimposed, the distal portion of the navicular projects along the volar aspect

Imaging Technique

Film size: 8 × 10" (2 × 13 × 18 cm), crosswise (divided; one-half covered with a lead mask for two projections) or 18 × 24 cm, crosswise (divided for four projections)
Film speed: 100
FFD: 40" (100 cm)
Bucky: no (tabletop technique)
Focal spot: small
Manual exposure: 44–46 kV; 8–16 mAs,   …mAs,   …mAs

Patient Preparation

— Remove everything from the forearm
— Remove jewelry (ring, watch)

Positioning

— Patient sits at the side of the table (legs *not* under the table)
— Forearm resting on the table, immobilized with a sandbag
Navicular bone, position I
— Wrist rests with the inferior surface on the middle of the cassette
— Hand in extreme ulnar flexion (thumb and radius form a straight line)
— The metacarpophalangeal joints are extended, interphalangeal joints are flexed
Navicular bone, position II
— Palmar surface of the hand turned down
— Radial side elevated 45° (thumb up), 2nd to the 5th fingers slightly abducted to the ulnar side, supported with a sponge wedge
Navicular bone, position III
— Palmar surface of the hand turned down
— Ulnar side elevated 45° (little finger up), 2nd to the 5th fingers slightly abducted to the ulnar side, supported with a sponge wedge
Navicular bone, position IV
— Palmar surface of the hand rests flat on a 15° sponge wedge
— Fingers slightly abducted to the ulnar side or
Navicular bone, position IV (variation)
— Wrist in true lateral position, ulnar side resting on the middle of the cassette
— Hand hyperextended in dorsiflexion, loose fist
— Gonads shielded (lead apron)

Navicular bone, position I

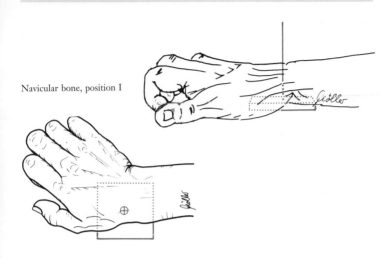

Navicular bone, position II

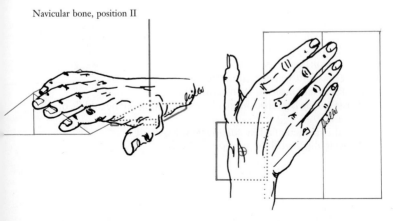

Alignment
— Projection: dorsovolar, perpendicular to the film
— Central ray directed to the navicular bone (or in variation IV to the center of the wrist and middle of the film)
— Centering, collimation, side identification

Tips & Tricks
— Lateral collimation on the ulnar side not more than to midwrist
— Use magnifying technique (e.g., for fractures) (increased object-to-film distance, 0.3 mm smallest focal spot)

Navicular bone, position III

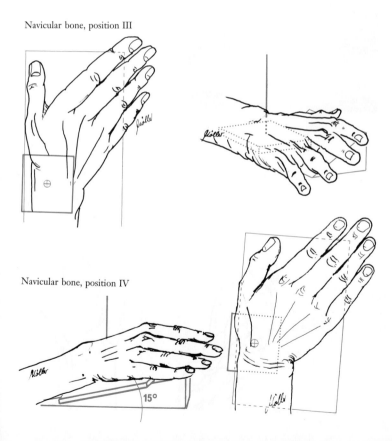

Navicular bone, position IV

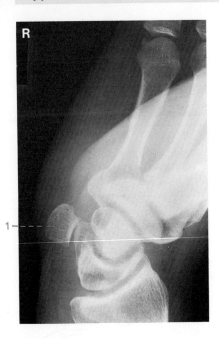

■ **Criteria of a Good Radiographic View**
Clear projection of the pisiform bone (1)

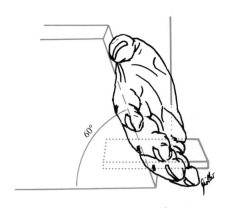

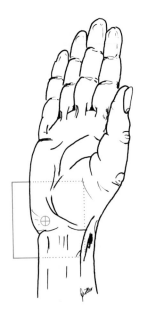

Imaging Technique

Film size: 8 × 10" (13 × 18 cm or 18 × 24 cm), lengthwise
Film speed: 100
FFD: 40" (100 cm)
Bucky: no (tabletop technique)
Focal spot: small
Manual exposure: 40–50 kV; 16–20 mAs,   …mAs,   …mAs

Patient Preparation

— Remove everything from the forearm
— Remove jewelry (ring, watch)

Positioning

— Patient sits at the table, placing the dorsum of the hand on the table
— Radial side (thumb up) elevated 60°
— Supported with sponge wedges (for instance, a 15° and a 45° wedge)
— Gonads shielded (large lead apron)

Alignment

— Projection: oblique radiodorsal, perpendicular to the film
— Central ray directed to the pisiform bone and to the middle of the film
— Centering, collimation, side identification

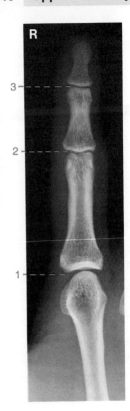

Criteria of a Good Radiographic View

Metacarpophalangeal (1), proximal (2), and distal (3) interphalangeal joints with no superimposition

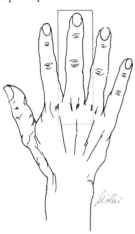

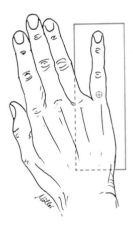

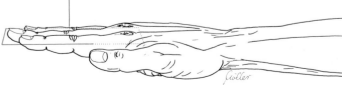

Imaging Technique
Film size: 8 × 10" (13 × 18 cm), lengthwise (divided; one-half covered with lead mask)
Film speed: 100
FFD: 40" (100 cm)
Bucky: no (tabletop technique)
Focal spot: small
Manual exposure: 44 kV; 6.4 mAs,   …mAs,   …mAs

Patient Preparation
— Remove everything from the forearm
— Remove jewelry (ring, watch)

Positioning

— Patient sits at the side of the table
— Hand rests with the palmar surface on the cassette
— Finger being examined centered to the midline of the (unmasked half) of the cassette
— The other fingers abducted
— Gonads shielded (lead apron)

Alignment
— Projection: dorsovolar, perpendicular to the film
— Central ray directed to the proximal interphalangeal (or to the metacarpophalangeal joint, the part of the finger in question = central ray) and to the middle of the cassette
— Sandbag placed over the forearm
— Centering, collimation, side identification

Tips & Tricks
If the volar side of the finger is injured, place the dorsal sid eon the film, or use some gauze padding.

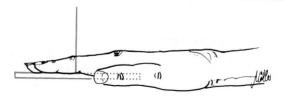

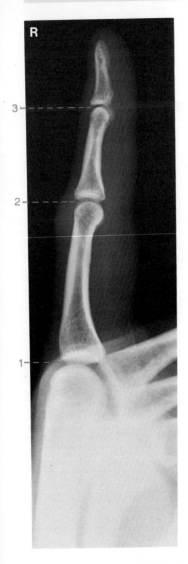

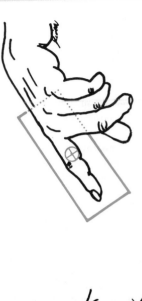

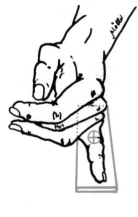

■ **Criteria of a Good Radiographic View**
Metacarpophalangeal (1), proximal (2), and distal (3) interphalangeal joints with no superimposition and in true lateral projection

Imaging Technique

Film size: 8 × 10" (13 × 18 cm), lengthwise (divided; one-half covered with lead mask)
Film speed: 100
FFD: 40" (100 cm)
Bucky: no (tabletop technique)
Focal spot: small
Manual exposure: 44 kV; 6–8 mAs,   …mAs,   …mAs

Patient Preparation

— Remove everything from the forearm
— Remove jewelry (ring, watch)

Positioning

— Patient sits at the side of the table (legs *not* under the table)
— Second and 3rd fingers rest on the cassette with their radial side, 4th and 5th fingers with their ulnar side (fingernails straight lateral, 3rd and 4th fingers supported so that the long axis of the entire finger is parallel to the film)
— Adjacent fingers flexed (use bands if necessary)
— Gonads shielded (large lead apron)

Alignment

— Projection: lateral (2nd and 3rd fingers ulnoradial, 4th and 5th fingers radioulnar), perpendicular to the film
— Central ray to the proximal IP joint and middle of the cassette
— Centering, collimation, side identification

Tips & Tricks

Immobilize the extended finger with a tongue depressor or hold with the fingers of the other hand.

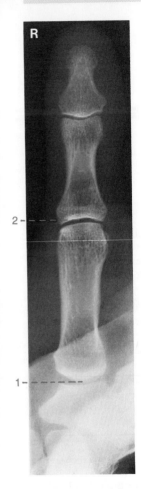

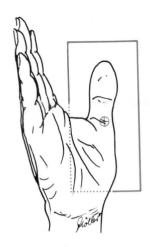

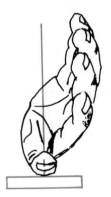

■ **Criteria of a Good Radiographic View**
Carpometacarpal joint (1) and thumb from the metacarpophalangeal
joint (2) to the tip with no superimposition

Imaging Technique

Film size: 8 × 10" (13 × 18 cm), crosswise (divided; one-half covered with a lead mask)
Film speed: 100
FFD: 40" (100 cm)
Bucky: no
Focal spot: small
Manual exposure: 44 kV, 8 mAs,   …mAs,   …mAs

Patient Preparation

— Remove everything from the forearm
— Remove jewelry (ring, watch)

Positioning

— Patient sits at the side of the table (legs *not* under the table)
— Forearm in maximal internal rotation
— Dorsum of the thumb and metacarpal are resting directly on the cassette
— Maximal pronation, dorsum of the hand supported on a sponge wedge
— Gonads shielded (large lead apron)

Alignment

— Projection: volodorsal, perpendicular to the film
— Central ray directed to the metacarpophalangeal joint of the thumb and the middle of the cassette
— Centering, collimation, side identification

Tips & Tricks

— The film can also be taken at the upright bucky stand (cassette centered on the affected part, the arm adducted and flexed, hand rotated inward, dorsum of the thumb placed on the cassette and immobilized)
— If internal rotation is not possible: patient places the hand in a lateral position with the little finger (ulnar) side down, thumb is abducted and placed on the (elevated and supported) cassette
— Sometimes positioning may be more comfortable for the patient if the arm is abducted dorsally (which means that the patient sits with the back to the table. Attention to gonad shielding!)

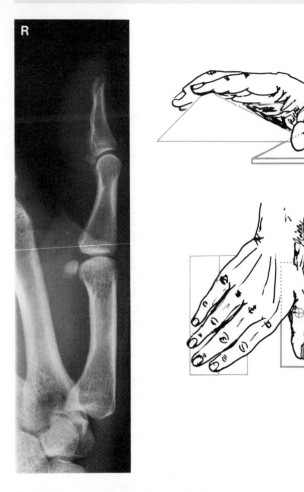

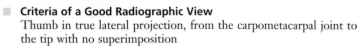

■ **Criteria of a Good Radiographic View**
Thumb in true lateral projection, from the carpometacarpal joint to the tip with no superimposition

Imaging Technique
Film size: 8 × 10" (13 × 18 cm), crosswise (divided; one-half covered with lead mask)
Film speed: 100
FFD: 40" (105 cm)
Bucky: no
Focal spot: small
Manual exposure: 44 kV; 8 mAs,   …mAs,   …mAs

Patient Preparation
— Remove everything from the forearm
— Remove jewelry (ring, watch)

Positioning
— Patient sits at the side of the table (legs *not* under the table)
— The abducted thumb rests with the radial side on the cassette (fingernail straight lateral)
— The other four fingers are elevated and supported on a sponge wedge
— Gonads shielded (lead apron)

Alignment
— Projection: lateral (ulnoradial), perpendicular to the film
— Central ray directed to the metacarpophalangeal joint of the thumb and middle of the cassette
— Centering, collimation, side identification

Variations
— With a lossely closed fist (hand arched) and the thumb abducted, the thumb is in a lateral position that requires no sponge support
— Oblique view of the thumb: when the hand lies flat, the thumb is in an oblique position, alignment otherwise as above

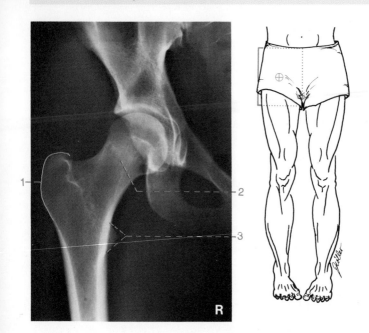

Criteria of a Good Radiographic View
— Complete visualization of the hip joint (from the lower portion of the iliac wing to the proximal femur)
— Hip joint in the upper third of the film
— Greater trochanter (1) forms the lateral margin (should not be superimposed on the femoral neck)
— Femoral neck not foreshortened (2)
— Lesser trochanter forms the inner margin (3)

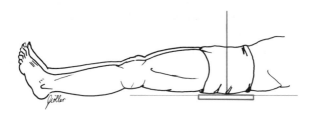

Imaging Technique
Film size: 10 × 12" (24 × 30 cm), lengthwise
Film speed: 200 (400)
FFD: 40" (115 cm)
Bucky: yes (under the table)
Focal spot: large
Exposure: 70–77 kV, automatic, center cell

Patient Preparation
— Remove clothes from the waist down, except underwear

Positioning

— Supine, legs straight (parallel to the longitudinal axis of the body)
— Feet turned inward (large toes touching) (no internal rotation if a fracture is suspected)
— Gonads shielded

Alignment
— Projection: AP, perpendicular to the film
— Central ray to the center of the femoral neck (midinguinal) and the middle of the cassette
— Upper border of the cassette: anterior superior iliac spine
— Centering, collimation, side identification (inferior, lateral)
— Breathing suspended after expiration

Variation
If there is a prosthetic device present
— Use a larger film size (7 × 17" [20 × 40 cm])
— Don't use photocell

Tips & Tricks
— the femoral artery pulse can be used as a centering aid; it is located over the femoral head
— Put a sandbag across the lower leg

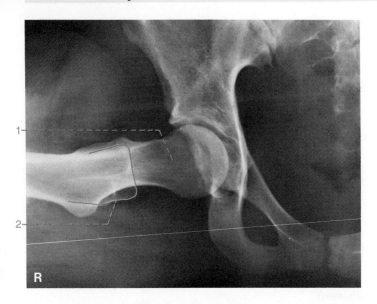

R

■ **Criteria of a Good Radiographic View**
   — Complete visualization of the hip joint
   — Femoral neck and shaft in straight alignment (1)
   — The greater trochanter (2) is partly projected behind the femoral neck

Imaging Technique
Film size: 10 × 12" (24 × 30 cm), lengthwise
Film speed: 200
FFD: 40" (115 cm)
Bucky: yes (under the table)
Focal spot: large
Exposure: 77 kV, automatic, center cell

Patient Preparation
— Remove clothes from the waist down, except underwear

Positioning

— Supine position
— The affected hip joint in 45° flexion and 45° abduction
— Thigh supported on padding
— Gonads shielded (lead apron, testicle cups)

Alignment
— Projection: AP, perpendicular to the film
— Central ray directed to the center of the femoral neck (midinguinal) and the middle of the cassette (anterior superior iliac spine at the upper border of the cassette)
— Centering, collimation, side identification
— Breathing suspended after expiration

Variations
Lauenstein I
— Supine position, hip and knee flexed 45°
— Opposite side elevated until the affected hip is in a lateral position
Lauenstein II
— Supine position, hip and knee flexed so that the sole of the foot stands on the table
— Leg slightly abducted (bent outward), not rotated externally
— Central ray 2FB lateral to and above the inguinal midpoint

(Page 157 cont.)

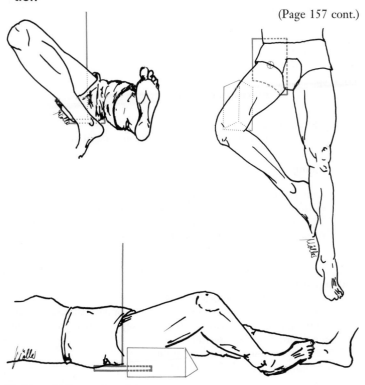

Hip joint, axial, Lauenstein projetion

Tips & Tricks

— If the patient's ability to move is limited, elevate and support the unaffected side

— Put the cassette diagonally into the table tray (angle the tube accordingly) = better positioning, shows more of the femur (the femur projects into the lower lateral corner of the cassette)

— If a prosthetic device is present, a larger cassette (e.g., 7 × 17" [18 × 43 cm]) may be required

Imaging Technique
Film size: 10 × 12" (24 × 30 cm), lengthwise
Film speed: 200
FFD: 40" (115 cm)
Bucky: yes (under the table)
Focal spot: large
Exposure: 77 kV, automatic, center cell

Patient Preparation
— Remove clothes from the waist down, except underwear

Positioning

— Supine position
— 1. Hip joint to be examined flexed 45° (30°–60°), foot stands on the table
— 2. Hip joint to be examined extended, foot in slight internal rotation
— Upper border of the cassette at the level of the anterior superior iliac spine
— Gonads shielded (lead apron, testicle cup)

Alignment
— Projection:
   1. AP, perpendicular to the film
   2. 30° craniocaudad angulation
— Central ray directed to the center of the femoral neck (midinguinal) and middle of the cassette
— Centering, collimation, side identification

Variations
Faux-profile view
— Patient stands sideways with the affected hip turned towards the vertical bucky stand
— Foot on the affected side parallel to the stand
— The pelvic half away from the film is rotated back at a 65° angle toward the stand (the healthy leg included)
— Arms above the head
— Central ray directed perpendicularly to the hip to be examined (about 2 FB medial to the inguinal midpoint)

(continued on pp. 160, 161)

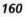

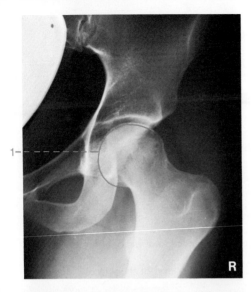

View 1:
Anterior contour

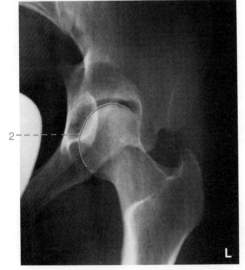

View 2:
Posterior contour

Criteria of a Good Radiographic View
— Joint space in the center of the film
— Contour of the femoral head outlined (1 = anterior, 2 = posterior contour)

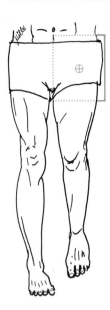

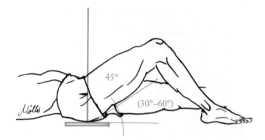

1. Contour view of the femoral head
(anterior contour)

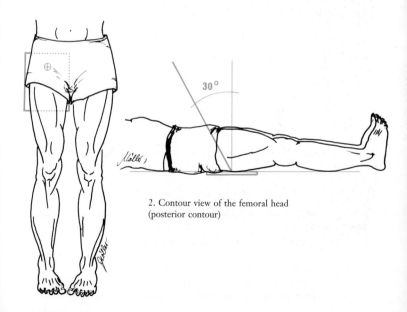

2. Contour view of the femoral head
(posterior contour)

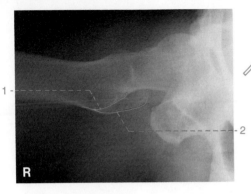

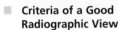

- ### Criteria of a Good Radiographic View
  — Complete visualization of the hip joint
  — Femoral neck in the center of the film, unforeshortened and without superimposition
  — Trochanters projected "underneath" (1 and 2)

Alignment
  — Projection: oblique, about 45°, from caudomedial to craniolateral, perpendicular to the film
  — Central ray directed to the center of the femoral neck (midinguinal)
  — Centering, collimation side identification

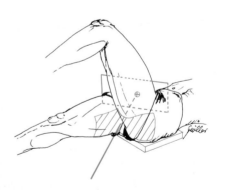

Tips & Tricks
  — Cassette must be placed well inside the waist
  — Buttocks supported so that the femoral neck is centered over the midpoint of the film
  — If no screen is being used, place bags with rice flour on the inside of the thigh to compensate for differences in density

Imaging Technique
Film size: 10 × 12" (24 × 30 cm), lengthwise
Film speed: 200 (if screen is used, +towards the hip)
FFD: 40" (100 cm)
Bucky: grid cassette, tabletop technique
Focal spot: large
Manual exposure: 85 kV; 80 mAs,   …mAs,   …mAs

Patient Preparation
— Remove clothes from the waist down, except underwear

Positioning

— Supine position, buttocks supported (elevated)
— Hip joint to be examined is extended, rotated medially by perhaps 10° (not when a fracture is present)
— The healthy leg is completely flexed at the hip (and knee joint) and elevated (for instance, on a wooden box)
— The cassette is placed upright against the outside of the affected hip, perpendicular to the plane of the table and parallel to the femoral neck (at an angle of about 45° toward the longitudinal axis), and is supported in the vertical position with a sandbag or wedge pillow

Variations
Hips in sitting position, semiaxial projection
— Patient seated with the back to the vertical bucky stand (on a wooden box, for instance), pelvis adjacent to the cassette tray
  Both thighs abducted exactly 20° each from the median sagittal plane
— Film size: 7 × 17" (20 × 40 or 18 × 43 cm)
— Film speed: 400
— Bucky: yes (upright bucky stand)
— Exposure: 80 kV, automatic, center cell
  (lower cassette border 1–2 cm below the seat level)
Antetorsion view of the hips, Rippstein position
— Patient in supine position, leg-holder device brought up to the pelvis
— Legs placed on the holder in such a way that hip and knee are flexed at right angles and both hips are abducted 20° each from the median sagittal plane
— Otherwise same as the sitting view

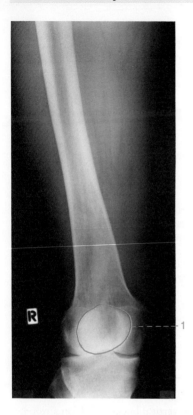
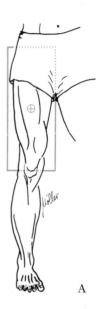

A

■ **Criteria of a Good Radiographic View**
— Femur exactly AP
— Hip joint (greater trochanter forms the lateral border) or knee joint (patella [1] overlying the middle of the femur) are included in the view

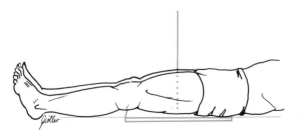

B

Imaging Technique

Film size: 7 × 17" (20 × 40 or 18 × 43 cm), lengthwise
Film speed: 200, compensating screen +/– (+ = on top)
FFD: 40" (115 cm)
Bucky: yes
Focal spot: large
Exposure: 70 kV, automatic, center cell

Patient Preparation

— Remove clothes from the waist down, except underwear

Positioning

— Supine position
— Legs straight, slightly rotated medially
— Opposite leg somewhat abducted
  Either
A. *(with hip joint)*
— Upper cassette border at the anterior superior iliac spine or
B. *(with knee joint)*
— Lower cassette border about 5 cm below the joint space of the knee
— Gonads shielded (lead apron)

Alignment

— Projection: AP, perpendicular to the film
— Central ray directed to the middle of the cassette
— Centering, collimation, side identification
— Breathing suspended after expiration

Variation

Femur, with both joints
— Film size: 20 × 60 cm
— Upper border: anterior superior iliac spine

Tips & Tricks

— Use either a wedge filter or rice flour to compensate for density differences
— Adjustment of the longitudinal axis of the leg is best done from the foot
— Maintain and immobilize the rotation by placing a sandbag across the lower leg

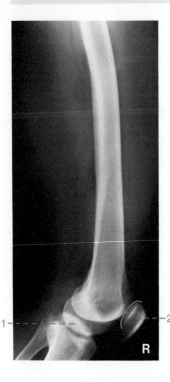

- **Criteria of a Good Radiographic View**
  — Femur straight lateral
  — Hip or knee joint (1) included on the film
  — Patella clearly shown (2) (on film that includes the knee joint)

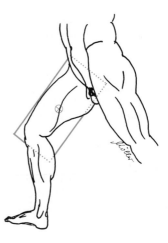

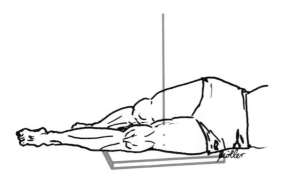

Imaging Technique

Film size: 7 × 17" (8 × 43 or 20 × 40 cm), lengthwise
Film speed: 200, compensating screen +/–
FFD: 40" (115 cm)
Bucky: yes (under the table)
Focal spot: large
Exposure: 70–80 kV for the hip; 60–65 kV for the knee joint, automatic, center cell

Patient Preparation

— Remove clothes from the waist down, except underwear

Positioning

— Patient lies on the side, the leg to be examined is placed in lateral position on the table, hip and knee flexed
— The other leg either:
  A. (Femur, including hip joint) hyperextended and placed behind the leg to be examined (upper cassette border [+] at the level of the anterior superior iliac spine)
  or
  B. (Femur, including knee joint) strongly flexed, supported, placed in front of the leg to be examined (lower cassette border [–] about 5 cm below the joint space of the knee)
— Gonads shielded (testicle cups for men)

Alignment

— Projection: mediolateral, perpendicular to the film
— Central ray directed to the middle of the cassette (which is centered in A over the proximal, in B over the distal third of the femur)
— Centering, collimation, side identification
— Breathing suspended after expiration

Variation

View of the femur with both joints:
— Film size: 20 × 60 cm
— Upper cassette border at the level of the anterior superior iliac spine, otherwise as in A

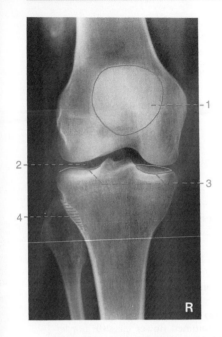

■ **Criteria of a Good Radiographic View**
— Patella in midline (1)
— Joint space clearly defined (2)
— Planar projection of the tibial plateau
— Tibia superimposed on the medial aspect
 of the fibular head only

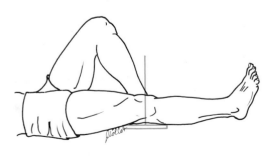

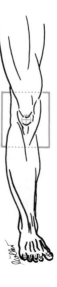

Imaging Technique

Film size: 8 × 10" (18 × 24 cm), lengthwise (or 10 × 12" [24 × 30 cm], crosswise, divided for two views)
Film speed: 200
FFD: 40" (115 or 100 cm)
Bucky: yes (no)
Focal spot: small
Exposure:
— bucky tray under the table: 60–70 kV, automatic, center cell
— tabletop technique without bucky: 50–55 kV; 25–30 mAs, …mAs, …mAs

Patient Preparation

— Remove clothes from the waist down, except underwear

Positioning

— Supine position, leg extended, in slight internal rotation (until patella is in midline)
— Other leg abducted
— Lower leg immobilized with sandbag
— Gonads shielded (large lead apron)

Alignment

— Projection: AP, perpendicular to the film
— Central ray directed to the midpoint of the joint space (2 cm = 1 FB below the superior pole of the patella) and middle of the cassette
— Centering, collimation, side identification

Tips & Tricks

— If the knee cannot be fully extended, support the knee, then move the central ray distally about 1 or 2 cm
— Increase the focal film distance to lessen magnification (exposure correction for manual setting: 1 exposure point for every 10 cm)
— If cruciate ligament injury is suspected, have the patient slightly bend the knee to demonstrate the intercondylar tubercles

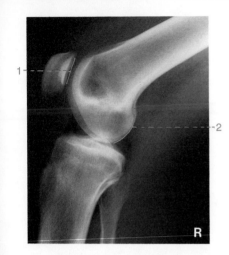

■ **Criteria of a Good Radiographic View**
— Posterior surface of the patella clearly delineated (1)
— Femoral condyles superimposed (especially dorsal aspect, 2)
— Joint space of the knee clearly visualized
— Tibial tuberosity can be evaluated

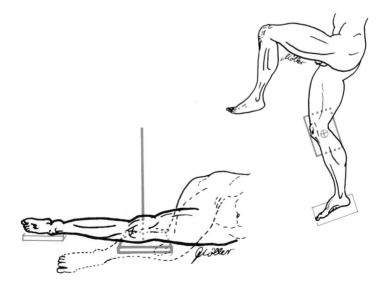

Imaging Technique

Film size: 8 × 10" (18 × 24 cm), lengthwise (or 10 × 12" [24 × 30 cm], crosswise; divided for two views)
Film speed: 200
FFD: 40" (115 or 100 cm)
Bucky: yes (no)
Focal spot: small
Exposure:
— bucky tray under the table: 60 kV, automatic, center cell
— tabletop technique without bucky: 55–55 kV; 25–30 mAs, …mAs, …mAs

Patient Preparation

— Remove clothes from the waist down, except underwear

Positioning

— Patient lies on side, the lateral side of the knee is placed on the cassette (or on the table)
— Knee flexed 30° to 45°
— Lower leg parallel to the surface plane (heel/calcaneus supported with a sponge)
— Opposite leg placed in front of the leg to be examined
— Gonads shielded (lead apron)

Alignment

— Projection: lateral, perpendicular to the film
— Central ray directed to the midpoint of the joint space (2 cm below the superior pole of the patella) and middle of the cassette
— Centering, collimation, side identification

Variation

If mobility is restricted, place the cassette upright on its edge and take the film in horizontal projection.

Tips & Tricks

— If there is osteoporosis, reduce the kilardtage (to about 55 kV)
— Don't make the films too dark, or soft-tissue changes may be missed

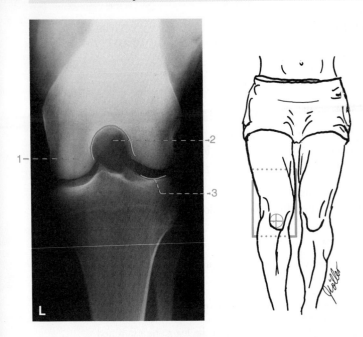

■ **Criteria of a Good Radiographic View**
— Joint space (intercondylar fossa) clearly defined (2)
— Femoral condyles with no superimposition (1)
— Linear projection of the lateral tibial plateau (3)

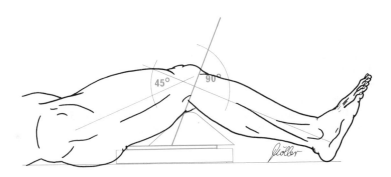

Imaging Technique
Film size: 8 × 10" (18 × 24 cm), lengthwise (curved cassette)
Film speed: 200
FFD: 40" (100 cm)
Bucky: no (tabletop technique)
Focal spot: small
Manual exposure: 50–60 kV; 25–32 mAs,   …mAs,   …mAs

Patient Preparation
— Remove clothes from the waist down, except underwear

Positioning

— Supine position
— A. Cassette is placed on a sponge pad and under a triangular sponge
   wedge
— The affected knee is put on the wedge and flexed 45°
— Patella in midline position (leg in slight internal rotation)
— The other leg is abducted
Or
— B. The curved cassette is put over the triangular wedge in the
   popliteal fossa
— Gonads shielded (lead apron)

Alignment
— Projection: perpendicular to the axis of the lower leg, (about
   30°–45° caudocephalad toward the film)
— Central ray directed to the midpoint of the joint space (2–3 cm
   below the lower pole of the patella) and the middle of the cassette
— Centering, collimation, side identification

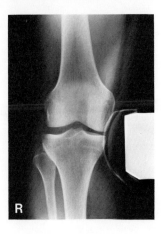

Criteria of a Good Radiographic View

AP view of the knee:
— Joint space freely visible
— Planar projection of the tibial plateau
— Tibia superimposed only on the medial aspect of the head of the fibula

Lateral view of the knee:
— Posterior surface of the patella clearly delineated
— Femoral condyles largely superimposed
— Joint space of the knee freely visible

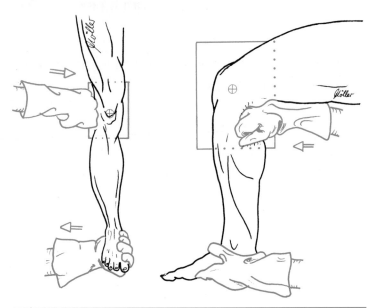

Alignment
— Projection: AP or lateral, perpendicular to the film
— Central ray directed to the midpoint of the joint space (2 cm = 1 FB below the superior pole of the patella and the middle of the cassette)
— Centering, collimation, side identification, notation of the applied pressure (15 kp)

Imaging Technique

Film size: 8 × 10" (18 × 24 cm), lengthwise, (or 10 × 12" [24 × 30 cm], crosswise, divided for two views)
Film speed: 200   FFD: 40" (115 or 100 cm)
Bucky: yes (no)   Focal spot: small
Exposure: with bucky tray under the table: 60–70 kV, automatic, center cell; tabletop technique without bucky: 50–55 kV; 25–30 mAs, …mAs,   …mAs

Patient Preparation

— Remove clothes from the waist down, except underwear
— Make certain that there is no fracture of the femur or lower leg (take a preliminary film if there are symptoms)

Positioning

A. Knee AP (to test the medial and lateral ligaments)
— With the patient seated, the leg is flexed 15°–30° (supported if necessary); the opposite leg is abducted
— The examiner, wearing lead apron and gloves, puts stress on the knee joint by applying lateral (or medial) traction on the foot, and with the other hand exerts pressure on the outside (or on the inside) of the knee joint
— If the restraining assembly is used, the pressure plate of the support is placed at the level of the joint space, exactly opposite the midpoint of the counter-pressure pad, and pressure is set at 15 kp
B. Lateral knee (to test the anterior and posterior cruciate ligaments)
— The patient lies on the affected side, with the lateral aspect of the knee down, knee flexed 90°. The examiner, wearing lead apron and gloves, holds the patient's leg parallel to the plane of the tabletop with one hand, and with the other hand (fist) exerts maximal pressure against the lower leg below the popliteal fossa ("anterior compartment"). When testing the anterior cruciate ligament ("posterior compartment"), the pressure is applied against the anterior surface of the lower leg while positioning remains otherwise the same
— When using restraining assembly, the knee is flexed 10°–20° when placed into the holder, and pressure to be applied is set at 15 kp

Tips & Tricks

— Always take both sides for comparison and make certain the force applied is equal
When using the restraining assembly:
— Recheck pressure settings shortly before taking the films
— When testing the anterior cruciate ligament of muscular athletic patients, the pressure applied should be increased to 20 kp

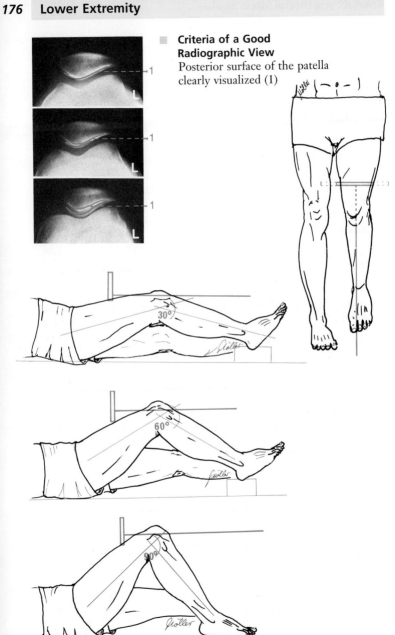

Criteria of a Good Radiographic View
Posterior surface of the patella clearly visualized (1)

Imaging Technique

Film size: 7 × 17" (18 × 43 cm), crosswise, divided for three views on one film
Film speed: 200
FFD: 40" (100 cm)
Bucky: no (tabletop technique)
Focal spot: small
Manual exposure: 50–60 kV; about 25 mAs,   …mAs,   …mAs

Patient Preparation

— Remove clothes from the waist down, except underwear

Positioning

— Patient seated on the examining table
— Leg flexed:
  1st view: 150° (30°), 2nd view: 120° (60°), 3rd view: 90° (90°)
  (angle of the longitudinal axis upper/lower leg)
— Patella parallel to the table
— Cassette placed upright on the thigh, perpendicular to the table
  (either in a cassette holder, or patients hold the cassette themselves)
— Upper border of the cassette = one hand's breadth above the patella
— Gonads shielded (lead apron)

Alignment

— Projection: horizontal caudocephalad (parallel to the patella)
— Central ray directed to the midpoint of the lower border of the patella, perpendicular to the middle of the cassette
— Centering, collimation, side identification

Variation

Patella, axial projection, Settegast position
— Prone position, thigh rests on the table, and the anterior knee on the cassette
— Lower leg flexed until upper and lower leg form an angle of 45°
— Projection and central ray as above

Tips & Tricks

For help with positioning, place cardboard cutouts (30°, 60°, 90°) at the side of the knee.

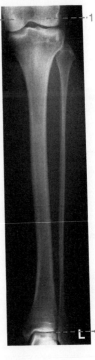

Criteria of a Good Radiographic View
— Lower leg in straight AP projection
— Knee or ankle joint included on the film
— Femoral condyles form the lateral margins, patella superimposed on midfemur (1)
— Ankle joint clearly visualized (2)

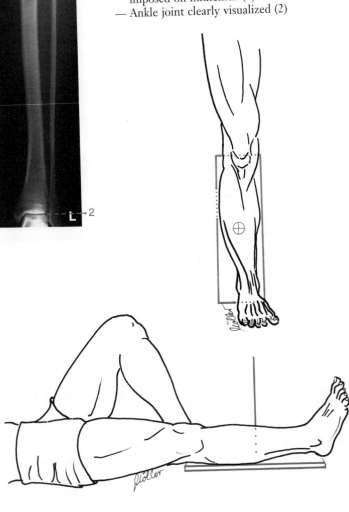

Imaging Technique
Film size: 7 × 17" (18 × 43 cm), lengthwise (or 14 × 17" [30 × 40 cm],
divided; 7 × 17" [with knee joint], 15 × 20 cm [with ankle joint], with +/−
compensating screen [+ towards the knee])
Film speed: 200
FFD: 40" (115 or 100 cm)
Bucky: yes (no)
Focal spot: small
Exposure:
— with bucky tray under the table: 60 kV, automatic, center cell
— tabletop technique without bucky:
   knee joint incl.: 50–55 kV; 25 mAs,   …mAs,   …mAs
   ankle joint incl: 50–55 kV; 5–8 mAs,   …mAs,   …mAs

Patient Preparation
— Remove clothes from the waist down, except underwear

Positioning

— Supine position, leg extended, slightly rotated medially:
A. with knee joint included: patella in frontal position
B. with ankle joint included: medial rotation, foot slightly dorsiflexed,
   opposite leg abducted
— Cassette:
A. with knee joint: upper cassette border 4 cm above joint space
B. lower cassette border at the plantar level
— Gonads shielded (large lead apron)

Alignment
— Projection: AP, perpendicular to the film
— Central ray directed to the middle of the cassette
— Centering, collimation, side identification

Tips & Tricks
— Put a bag with rice flour on the ankle joint and lower leg to com-
   pensate for density differences (compensating screen preferable)
— To get a truly straight view of the joint of interest, center to the
   joint and angle the central ray to include the full field size
— Maintain the rotation by immobilizing with a sand bag

Criteria of a Good Radiographic View
— Lower leg straight lateral
— Knee (1) or ankle joint (2) included on the film

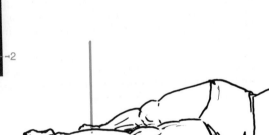

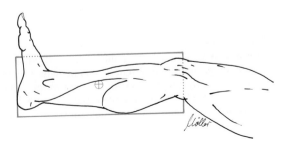

Imaging Technique

Film size: 7 × 17" (18 × 43 cm), lengthwise (or 14 × 17" [30 × 40 cm] divided; 20 × 40 cm [with knee joint], 15 × 20 cm [with ankle joint], with +/– compensating screen [+ towards the knee])
Film speed: 200
FFD: 40" (115 or 100 cm)
Bucky: yes (no)
Focal spot: small
Exposure:
— with bucky tray under the table: 55–60 kV, automatic, center cell
— tabletop technique without bucky:
   knee joint incl.: 50–55 kV; 25 mAs,   ...mAs,   ...mAs
   ankle joint incl.: 50–55 kV; 5–8 mAs,   ...mAs,   ...mAs

Patient Preparation
— Remove clothes from the waist down, except underwear

Positioning

— Patient lying on side, knee flexed about 30°
— Outside of the lower leg parallel to the cassette
— Opposite leg placed behind the leg to be examined
— Cassette:
A. with knee joint included: upper cassette border 4 cm above joint space, heel slightly supported
B. with ankle joint included: lower cassette border at plantar level, toes supported with a sponge wedge, foot slightly dorsiflexed
— Gonads shielded (large lead apron)

Alignment
— Projection: mediolateral, perpendicular to the film
— Central ray directed to the middle of the cassette
— Centering, collimation, side identification

Tips & Tricks
— Lateral position: lateral and medial malleolus in one plane
— Use compensating screen or rice flour, if necessary
— Take oblique views in 45° rotation, both medial and lateral

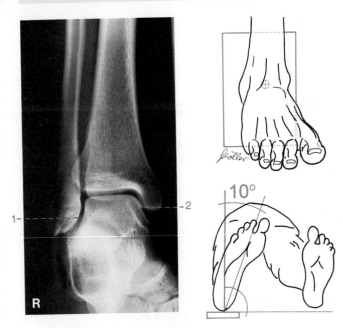

■ **Criteria of a Good Radiographic View**
— Ankle joint completely visualized, including medial and lateral malleoli and distal fibula
— Joint space between the medial malleolus and the talus (inside, 2), and between the lateral malleolus and the talus (outside, 1) clearly visible

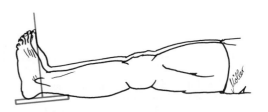

Imaging Technique

Film size: 8 × 10" (18 × 24 cm), crosswise, divided for two views
Film speed: 200
FFD: 40" (100 cm)
Bucky: no (tabletop technique)
Focal spot: small
Manual exposure: 50–60 kV; 20 mAs,   …mAs,   …mAs

Patient Preparation

— Uncover the lower leg

Positioning

— Supine position, leg extended, foot slightly rotated medially, about 10°–15°
— Foot dorsiflexed (plantar surface of the foot at a 90° angle with the lower leg)
— Opposite leg abducted
— Gonads shielded (lead apron)

Alignment

— Projection: AP, perpendicular to the film
— Central ray directed to the midpoint of the ankle joint (1 cm above the tip of the medial malleolus) and middle of the cassette
— Centering, collimation, side identification

Tips & Tricks

— Check medial rotation of the foot by aligning the little toe with the center of the ankle joint
— Malleolar mortise parallel to the film (and at equal distance from the cassette)

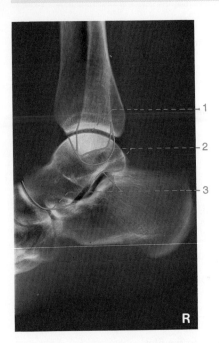

■ Criteria of a Good Radiographic View

— Ankle joint (1) and talocalcaneonavicular joint (3) in true lateral projection (malleoli superimposed [2] on each other)
— Calcaneus and talus completely included in the view
— Fibula is projected over the middle to distal third of the tibial joint surface

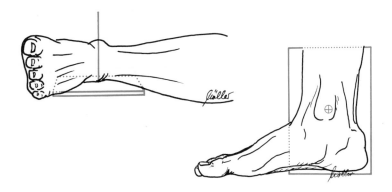

Imaging Technique
Film size: 8 × 10" (18 × 24 cm) crosswise, divided for two views (or 8 × 10", lengthwise)
Film speed: 200
FFD: 40" (100 cm)
Bucky: no (tabletop technique)
Focal spot: small
Manual exposure: 50–55 kV; 10–16 mAs,   …mAs,   …mAs

Patient Preparation
— Uncover the lower leg

Positioning

— Lateral position, the leg to be examined resting with the lateral malleolus close to the film
— Foot slightly dorsiflexed (lower leg/plantar surface = 90°)
— Straight lateral (malleoli exactly superimposed on each other)
— Flat sponge wedge put under the forefoot
— Healthy leg abducted
— Gonads shielded (large lead apron)

Alignment
— Projection: mediolateral, perpendicular to the film
— Central ray directed to the center of the ankle joint (midpoint of the medial malleolus) and middle of the cassette
— Centering, collimation, side identification

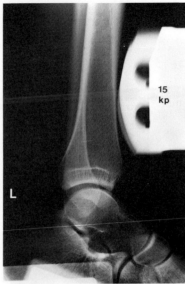

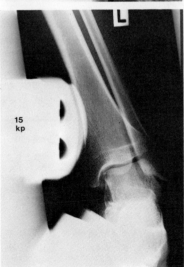

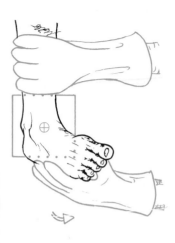

Criteria of a Good Radiographic View
— Ankle joint completely visualized, including both medial and lateral malleoli
— Clear view of the joint mortise

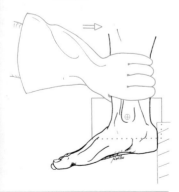

Tips & Tricks
— Always take both sides for comparison
— Make certain that the force applied is equal on both sides
When using the restraining assembly:
— Recheck pressure settings shortly before taking the films

Imaging Technique
Film size: 8 × 10" (18 × 24 cm), crosswise, divided for two views
Film speed: 200
FFD: 40" (100 cm)
Bucky: no (tabletop technique)
Focal spot: small
Manual exposure: 50–60 kV, 20 mAs,   …mAs,   …mAs

Patient Preparation
— Uncover the lower leg
— Rule out fracture (take a preliminary film if necessary)

Positioning

A. Like AP ankle (to test the medial and lateral ligaments)
— Patient supine, foot extended, the opposite leg abducted. The examiner, wearing lead apron and gloves, steadies the lower leg near the ankle joint with one hand while forcing the posterior foot into supination (or pronation) with the other hand
— If the restraining assembly is used, the pressure plate of the support is placed 1 FB above the medial (or lateral) malleolus, and pressure is set at 15 kp
B. Like lateral ankle (to test the anterior ligamentous support of the talus)
— Patient supine, foot turned inward about 15°, heel elevated on a board. While taking the film, the examiner, wearing lead apron and gloves, applies forceful pressure to the lower leg against the tabletop
— When using the restraining assembly, patient lies on the side, lateral side of the foot down, and foot slightly dorsiflexed (lower leg /plantar surface = 90°). Pressure plate of the support is placed against the anterior tibia 2–3 FB above the medial malleolus. Set pressure at 15 kp, then wait 1 min before taking the film

Alignment
— Projection: AP or lateral, perpendicular to the film
— Central ray directed to the midpoint of the ankle joint (1 cm above the tip of the medial malleolus) and to the middle of the cassette
— Centering, collimation, side identification, notation of applied pressure (15 kp)

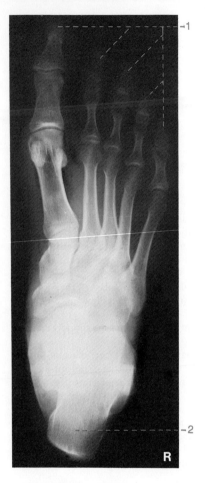

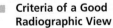

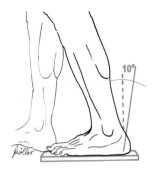

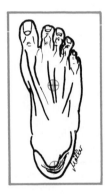

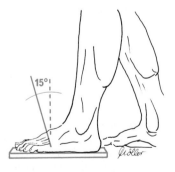

▦ **Criteria of a Good Radiographic View**
— Entire foot included, from the terminal phalanges (1) to the calcaneus (2) with no superimposition
— Good exposure

Imaging Technique
Film size: 10 × 12" (24 × 30 cm) lengthwise
Film speed: 100 (200) (possibly –/+ cassette)
FFD: 40" (100 cm)
Bucky: no (tabletop technique)
Focal spot: small
Manual exposure:
1. 50 kV; (8–10 mAs),   …mAs,   …mAs
2. 46 kV;   …mAs,   …mAs,   …mAs

Patient Preparation
— Remove clothes from the waist down, except underwear

Positioning

— Patient stands erect with the foot placed firmly on the cassette, which lies on the floor; foot immobilized on the cassette
— View 1: affected foot extended back as far as possible at the ankle joint, the opposite foot is placed for support behind the cassette, hands may grasp the armrest of a chair for additional support
— View 2: foot (with the plantar surface unchanged in its position) is anteflexed at the ankle joint; the opposite foot is placed in front of the cassette; hands may be placed for support on the thigh of the same side
— Gonads shielded (lead apron: 1. in front, 2. behind)

Alignment
View 1
— Projection: 15° anterior oblique, dorsoplantar (or vertical)
— Central ray directed to the midfoot
View 2
— Projection: –10° posterior oblique, dorsoplantar
— Central ray directed to the midcalcaneus
— Centering, collimation, side identification

Tips & Tricks
— Use rice flour or a filter for compensation of differences in density (except where there is a possibility of PCP [primary chronic polyarthritis])

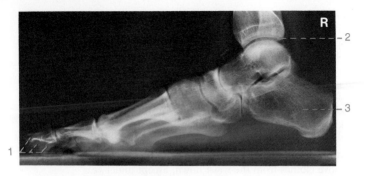

■ **Criteria of a Good Radiographic View**
  — Entire foot visible, including ankle joint (2), terminal phalanges (1), and calcaneus (3)
  — Lateral projection of the ankle joint (2)

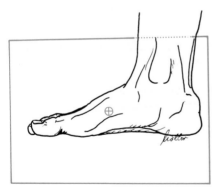

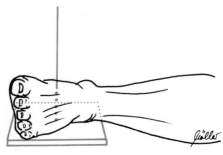

Imaging Technique
Film size: 10 × 12" (24 × 30 cm), crosswise
Film speed: 100 (200)
FFD: 40" (100 cm)
Bucky: no (tabletop technique)
Focal spot: small
Manual exposure: 50 kV; 10 mAs,   ...mAs,   ...mAs

Patient Preparation
— Uncover the foot (take off shoes, socks, pants)

Positioning

— Patient lies on side on the examining table, small-toe side on the film
— Midfoot centered over the film
— Heel elevated with sponge wedge
— Knee with suitable support
— Opposite leg placed anteriorly
— Gonads shielded (large lead apron)

Alignment
— Projection: mediolateral, perpendicular to the film
— Central ray directed to the midpoint of the foot and of the cassette
— Centering, collimation, side identification

Variations
— Examination may also be done with the patient standing up, a wooden block used for support, or in the supine position, a wooden block supporting the sole of the foot (at right angle to the axis of the lower leg)
— For small children, use a small board to dorsiflex the foot as far as possible (for club-foot demonstration)

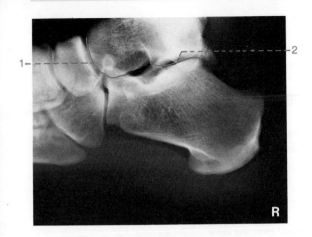

■ **Criteria of a Good Radiographic View**
 — True lateral projection
 — Calcaneus completely visualized
 — Talocalcaneonavicular joint (1 and 2) clearly
   demonstrated

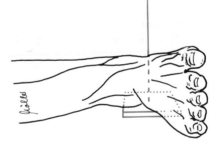

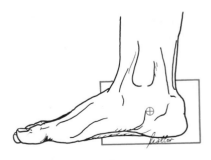

Imaging Technique

Film size: 8 × 10" (13 × 18 cm), crosswise (or 18 × 24 cm, crosswise, divided for two views)
Film speed: 100
FFD: 40" (100 cm)
Bucky: no (tabletop technique)
Focal spot: small
Manual exposure: 40–50 kV; 16–20 mAs,   …mAs,   …mAs

Patient Preparation

— Uncover thee foot (take off shoes, socks, pants)

Positioning

— Patient lies on side to be examined, lateral (small toe) side on the film
— Heel supported (elevated about 10°–15°)
— Leg flexed at the hip and knee
— The opposite leg placed anteriorly
— Heel centered over the cassette
— Gonads shielded (lead apron)

Alignment

— Projection: mediolateral, perpendicular to the film
— Central ray directed to the calcaneus (2–3 cm below and behind the medial malleolus) and to the center of the film
— Centering, collimation, side identification

Tips & Tricks

To evaluate the Achilles tendon (for possible rupture), use a softer beam (35–40 kV).

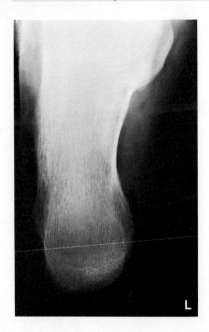

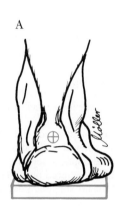

A

■ **Criteria of a Good Radiographic View**
   — Posterior aspect of the calcaneus clearly visible
   — Calcaneus complete and unforeshortened

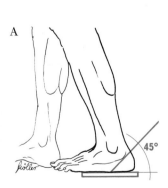

A

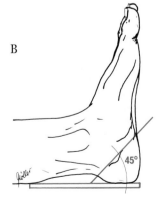

B

Imaging Technique
Film size: 8 × 10" (13 × 18 cm), lengthwise
Film speed: 100
FFD: 40" (100 cm)
Bucky: no (tabletop technique)
Focal spot: small
Manual exposure: 50–55 kV; 16–20 mAs,   …mAs,   …mAs

Patient Preparation
— Uncover the foot (take off shoes, socks, pants)

Positioning

— A. Patient places the foot on the cassette, foot flexed at the ankle joint
— B. Supine position, foot dorsiflexed (toes pulled with a band towards the lower leg as far as possible, foot and lower leg are in one plane = slight medial rotation), heel resting on the cassette (lower cassette border)
— Gonads shielded (large lead apron)

Alignment
— Projection: A. 45° oblique dorsoplantar
                    B. 45° oblique plantodorsal
— Central ray directed to the midpoint of the calcaneus and center of the film
— Centering, collimation, side identification

Tips & Tricks
Use rice flour to compensate for differences in density to provide good visualization of detail also of the anterior parts of the calcaneus, then use about 55 kV.

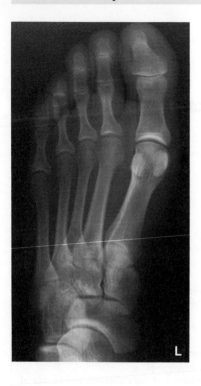

▨ **Criteria of a Good Radiographic View**
Complete view of the forefoot (and midfoot) without any superimposition

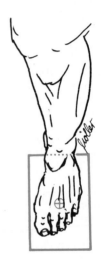

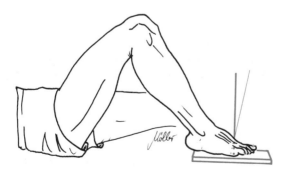

Imaging Technique
Film size: 8 × 10" (18 × 24 cm), crosswise, divided for two views
Film speed: 100
FFD: 40" (100 cm)
Bucky: no (tabletop technique)
Focal spot: small
Manual exposure: 44–48 kV; 8–10 mAs,   …mAs,   …mAs

Patient Preparation
— Uncover the foot (take off shoes, socks, pants)

Positioning

— Patient sits on the X-ray table, leg pulled up, forefoot and midfoot
  stand with their plantar surface on the cassette
— Gonads shielded (large lead apron)

Alignment
— Projection: perpendicular to the middle of the film (or 10° caudocephalad)
— Central ray directed to the head of the 3rd metatarsal (or to the
  midportion of the 3rd metatarsal if the midfoot is to be included)
  and to the center of the film
— Centering, collimation, side identification

Variation
View of the toes without any superimposition
— Film size: 8 × 10" (13 × 18 cm)
— Manual exposure: 40 kV; 8 mAs,   …mAs,   …mAs
— Otherwise as above
— Patient in prone position on the examining table
— The foot is rotated inward and rests with the back of the toes on the
  cassette
— supported with a sponge wedge

Tips & Tricks
— Use compensation filter or rice flour bag as needed
— Separate the toes with small rolled-up gauze pads or cotton balls

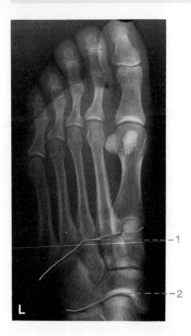

Criteria of a Good Radiographic View
— Complete visualization of the foorefoot and midfoot without any significant superimposition
— Clear demonstration of the Lisfranc (tarsometatarsal) (1) and Chopart (mediotarsal) (2) joints

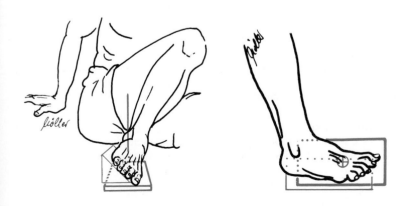

Imaging Technique

Film size: 10 × 12" (24 × 30 cm), crosswise, divided for two views
Film speed: 100 (200)
FFD: 40" (100 cm)
Bucky: no (tabletop technique)
Focal spot: small
Manual exposure:
— forefoot, oblique: 47 kV; 8–10 mAs,   …mAs,   …mAs
— foot (midfoot and forefoot), oblique: 47–55 kV; 13 mAs
— compensating filter if necessary

Patient Preparation

— Uncover the foot (take off shoes, socks, pants)

Positioning

— Patient sits on the X-ray table, leg drawn up, foot (forefoot) rests on the cassette
— Lower leg (and foot) adducted 45° (small-toe side elevated 45° and supported with a sponge wedge)
— Gonads shielded (large lead apron)

Alignment

— Projection: perpendicular to the middle of the film
— Central ray directed to, either
  (a) head of the 3rd metatarsal (forefoot) and middle of the film, or
  (b) midportion of the 3rd metatarsal (forefoot- and midfoot) and middle of the film
— Centering, collimation, side identification

Tips & Tricks

Separate the toes with small gauze pads.

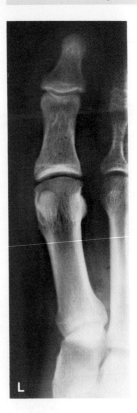

■ **Criteria of a Good Radiographic View**
Great toe completely visualized with no superimposition

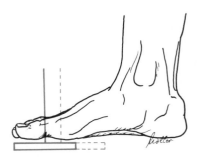

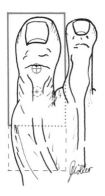

Imaging Technique
Film size: 8 × 10" (13 × 18 cm), lengthwise, divided for two views
Film speed: 100
FFD: 40" (100 cm)
Bucky: no (tabletop technique)
Focal spot: small
Manual exposure: 40–44 kV; 8 mAs,   …mAs,   …mAs

Patient Preparation
— Uncover the foot (take off shoes, socks)

Positioning

— Patient sits on the X-ray table, leg drawn up, the great toe rests flat on the cassette
— Padding (cotton) between the 1st and 2nd toes
— Gonads shielded (large lead apron)

Alignment
— Projection: dorsoplantar, perpendicular to the middle of the film
— Central ray directed to the MP joint of the great toe and middle of the film
— Centering, collimation to terminal phalanx or great toe, side identification

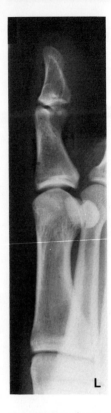

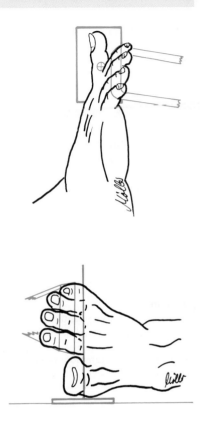

■ **Criteria of a Good Radiographic View**

Toe visualized in true lateral projection

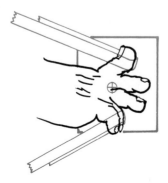

Imaging Technique

Film size: 8 × 10" (13 × 18 cm), lengthwise, divided for two views
Film speed: 100
FFD: 40" (100 cm)
Bucky: no (tabletop technique)
Focal spot: small
Manual exposure: 40 kV; 6,14–12 mAs,   …mAs,   …mAs

Patient Preparation

— Uncover the foot (take off shoes, socks)

Positioning

Toes 1–3
— Patient lies on the unaffected side, the great toe is placed laterally on the cassette
— (a) Great toe: the 2nd to 5th toes are pulled down with a band (srip of bandage)
— (b) Toes 2 and 3: the great toe is pulled up with a band, 4th and 5th toes are pulled down
Toes 4 and 5
— Patient lies on the affected side, the little toe is placed laterally on the cassette
— Either the toes 4 and 5 are elevated separately with a band each, or toes 1–3 are pulled up together
— Gonads shielded (lead apron)

Alignment

— Projection: mediolateral or lateromedial, perpendicular to the middle of the film
— Central ray directed to the metatarsophalangeal joint and midpoint of the film
— Centering, collimation, side identification

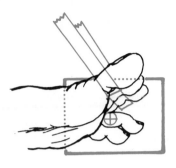

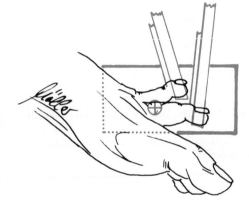

Other Non-Contrast Diagnostic Studies

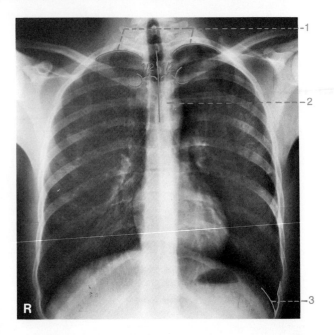

▨ Criteria of a Good Radiographic View
— Lungs fully visualized (costophrenic angle clearly seen, 3)
— Lateral sternum forms the anterior border (no ribs are projected in front of the sternum, 1)
— Posterior vertebral borders are plainly delineated (2)

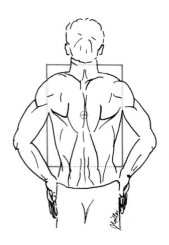
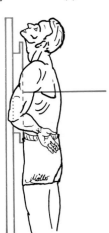

Imaging Technique
Film size: 14 × 17" (35 × 43 cm), lengthwise
Film speed: 200
FFD: 72" (180–200 cm)
Bucky: yes (under the table)
Focal spot: small (large in obese patients)
Exposure: 125 kV; automatic, all three cells (r. lateral cell)

Patient Preparation
— Remove all clothes from the waist up
— Take off jewelry (necklace, earrings)
— Have hair tied up on top of head

Positioning
— Patient stands with the chest facing the vertical cassette stand, leaning slightly forward
— Chest wall and both shoulders in contact with the cassette (patient lets the shoulders down)
— Hands placed on the hips, elbows rotated forward
— Head extended with the chin over the top of the cassette
— Upper cassette border 3 FB above the upper border of the shoulder
— Gonads shielded (lead apron)

Alignment
— Projection: dorsoventral (PA), perpendicular to the film
— Central ray directed to the spinal column at the level of the lower pole of the scapula
— Centering, collimation to the skin surface of the inferior costal arches, side identification
— Respiration suspended after deep inspiration

Variation
Chest in the recumbent position
— Manual exposure: 90–110 kV;   …mAs,   …mAs,   …mAs
— Bucky: 8/40 grid
If a pneumothorax is suspected: additional view after expiration

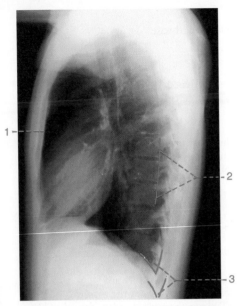

■ **Criteria of a Good Radiographic View**

— Lungs completely visualized (apices [1] and costophrenic angles [2] clearly visible)

— Symmetrical projection of the bony thorax (sternal ends of the clavicles equidistant from the spinous processes, thoracic spine in midline position [3])

— Sharp radiographic detail

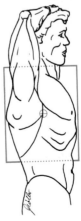

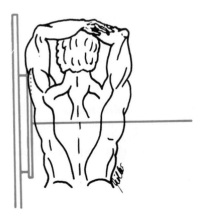

Imaging Technique
Film size: 14 × 17" (35 × 43 cm or 30 × 40 cm), lengthwise
Film speed: 200
FFD: 72" (200–180 cm)
Bucky: yes (under the table)
Focal spot: large
Exposure: 125 kV, automatic, center cell

Patient Preparation
— Remove all clothes from the waist up
— Take off jewelry (necklace, earrings)
— Have the hair tied up on top of head

Positioning

— Patient stands erect, with the left side against the film, straight lateral
— Arms extended upward above the head (or forehead, hands grasp the elbows)
— Upper body leans slightly forward
— Upper cassette border 3 FB above the upper border of the shoulder (vertebra prominens = 7th cervical vertebra)
— Gonads shielded (lead apron)

Alignment
— Projection: lateral, perpendicular to the film
— Central ray directed to the anterior axillary line at the level of the nipple (or tip the sternum)
— Centering, collimation, side identification

Variation
Right lateral view only in special diagnostic situations

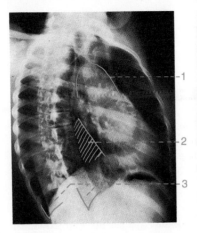 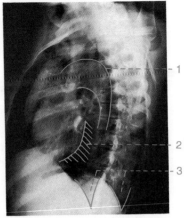

■ Criteria of a Good Radiographic View

A. Aortic arch foreshortened (1), retrocardiac space clearly visible (cardiac shadow projected away from the vertebral column, (2), esophagus demonstrated without any superimposition

B. Aortic arch uncoiled (1), retrocardiac space clearly visible (cardiac shadow projected away from the vertebral column, 2), lungs included from the apex to the costophrenic angle (3)

First oblique (RAO) position
(fencer position)

Second oblique (LAO) position
(boxer position)

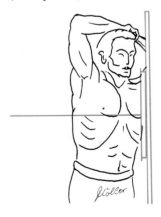 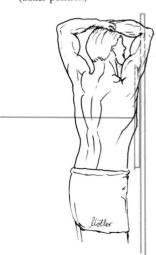

Imaging Technique
Film size: 14 × 17" (35 × 43 cm)
Film speed: 200
FFD: 72" (200–180 cm)
Bucky: yes (under the table, vertical bucky)
Focal spot: large
Exposure: 125 kV, automatic, all cells

Patient Preparation
— Remove all clothes from the waist up
— Take off jewelry (necklace, earrings)
— Have long hair tied up on top of head

Positioning

— A. First oblique (RAO, fencer position): patient stands at an oblique angle of 45° (to 60°) toward the plane of the film, right anterior chest wall in contact with the upright cassette
— B. Second oblique (LAO, boxer position): patient stands at an oblique angle of 45° (to 35°) toward the plane of the film, left anterior chest wall in contact with the upright cassette
— Arms raised above the head
— Upper border of the cassette 3 FB above the upper border of the shulder
— Gonads shielded (small lead apron)

Alignment
— Projection: oblique dorsoventral, perpendicular to the film
— Central ray directed to the vertebral column (not to the line of spinous processes but about one hand's breadth beside the processes) at the level of the inferior angle of the scapula
— Centering, collimation to skin border, side identification

Tips & Tricks
A contrast swallow may be used to outline the posterior cardiac border.

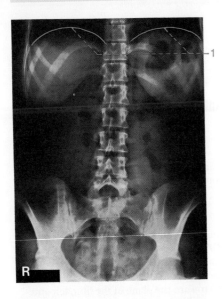

■ Criteria of a Good Radiographic View
Both domes of the diaphragm (1) and, as far as possible, the entire abdomen visualized completely and symmetrically

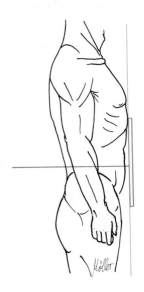

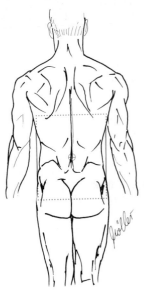

Imaging Technique

Film size: 14 × 17" (35 × 43 cm), lengthwise
Film speed: 400
FFD: 40" (115 cm)
Bucky: yes (under the table, vertical bucky)
Focal spot: large
Exposure: 117–125 kV, automatic, all cells

Patient Preparation

— Undress completely

Positioning

— Patient stands upright, the anterior abdomen against the vertical grid
— Upper cassette border at the level of the xiphoid process
— Gonads shielded (testicle cups for males)

Alignment

— Projection: dorsoventral, perpendicular to the film
— Central ray directed to the spinal column 2 cm above the iliac wing, middle of the cassette
— Collimation at least to the skin border or to 1 cm less than film size
— Side identification and "upright" marker
— Respiration suspended after expiration

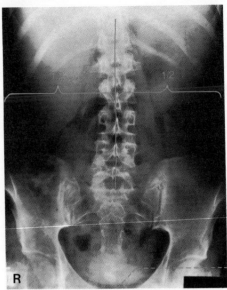

Criteria of a Good Radiographic View
— Upper border of the symphysis (1) demonstrated (also the domes of the diaphragms, if possible)
— Spinal column in midline position (2)

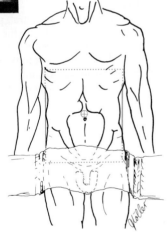

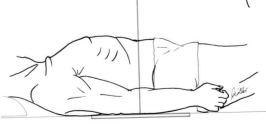

Imaging Technique
Film size: 14 × 17" (35 × 43 cm), lengthwise
Film speed: 400
FFD: 40" (115 cm)
Bucky: yes (under the table)
Focal spot: large
Exposure: 70 kV, automatic, all cells

Patient Preparation
— Undress completely

Positioning

— Supine position, arms along the sides of the body
— Lower cassette border 2 cm below the upper border of the symphysis
— Gonads shielded (testicle cups for men)

Alignment
— Projection: ventrodorsal, perpendicular to the film
— Central ray directed to midcassette in median plane, about 1 FB above the pelvic crest
— Lateral collimation to the anterior superior iliac spine on boths sides
— Side identification and "supine" marker
— Respiration suspended after expiration

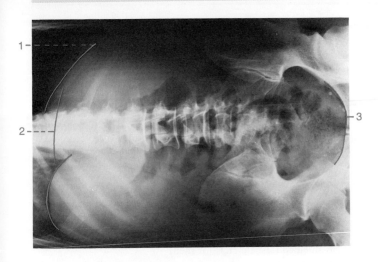

■ **Criteria of a Good Radiographic View**

— Correct exposure of the entire abdomen, especially of the right costophrenic space (1)

— The entire abdomen, from the diaphragms (2) to the upper border of the pubic symphysis (3), is included in the film

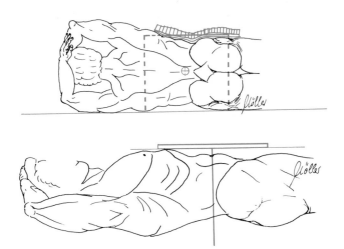

Imaging Technique
Film size: 14 × 17" (35 × 43 cm), lengthwise
Film speed: 400
FFD: 40" (115 cm)
Bucky: yes (vertical bucky grid)
Focal spot: large
Exposure: 117–125 kV, automatic, center cell (–1)

Patient Preparation
— Undress completely

Positioning

— Patient lies with the back (or abdomen in obese patients) against the cassette
— Arms placed above the head, legs slightly flexed for stabilization (patient must have been lying on the left side for at least 5 minutes to give possible free air time to rise)
— Upper border of the cassette 1 FB above the xiphoid process
— Respiration suspended after expiration
— Gonads shielded (testicle cups formen)

Alignment
— Projection: ventrodorsal (or dorsoventral), horizontal, perpendicular to the film
— Central ray directed to the spinal column 2 FB above the iliac crest and middle of the cassette
— Use of a filter to compensate for differences in density
— Collimation at least to the skin border, or to 1 cm less than film size
— side identification and marker "left decubitus"
— Respiration suspended after expiration

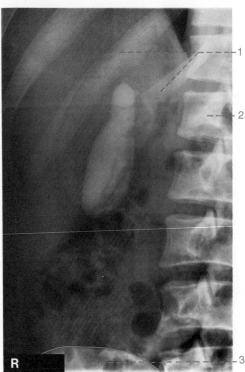

■ **Criteria of a Good Radiographic View**
— Lowest rib (1) and iliac crest (3) are both visualized
— Spinal column (2) projected along the film edge

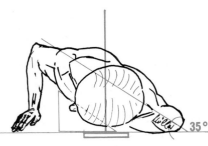

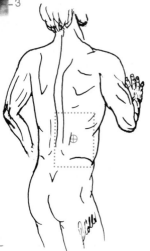

Imaging Technique

Film size: 10 × 12" (24 × 30 cm), lengthwise
Film speed: 200
FFD: 40" (115 cm)
Bucky: yes (under the table)
Focal spot: large
Exposure: 77 kV, automatic, center cell

Patient Preparation

— Undress, except underwear

Positioning

— Patient in the prone position, right side elevated about 35°
(20°–45°), supported with a sponge wedge (left arm along the side
of the body, the right arm used for support, knees slightly flexed for
additional stability)
— Right side of the body (midpoint between lowest rib and iliac crest)
centered over the cassette
— Gonads shielded

Alignment

— Projection: oblique ventrodorsal, perpendicular to the film
— Central ray directed to the middle of the cassette (about a hand's
breadth lateral to the spinous processes, at the midpoint between
the lowest rib and the iliac crest)
— Centering, lateral collimation to the skin border, side identification
— Respiration suspended after expiration

Variation

If tomographic films of the gallbladder are needed:
— 70 kV, medium thickness of the tomographic cuts, at a depth of
8–12 cm

Tips & Tricks

Mark the central ray on the skin with a skin marker (for later films or
corrections)
— Obese patient: gallbladder (and film center) more cranial and
lateral (20° elevation is sufficient)
— Thin patient: gallbladder (and film center) lower in the pelvis and
more medial (elevation of the right side up to 45°)

Criteria of a Good Radiographic View

— All of the breast tissues and axillary fold (1) are visualized, free of superimposed shadows (no skin folds) and sharply defined (without breathing motion)

— Nipple (2) in marginal profile (not projected over breast tissues)

— In the craniocaudad projection, the fatty tissues along the anterior thoracic wall should be seen as a dark line; in the mediolateral projection, the pectoral muscle should be visible as a light band of soft tissue density

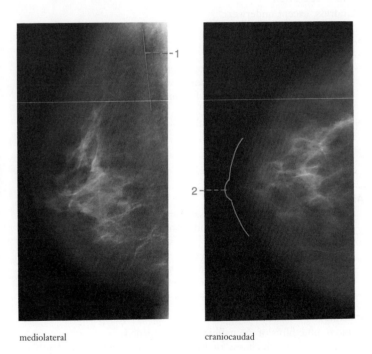

mediolateral   craniocaudad

Variation

Axillary projection: C-arm is rotated 45°. Otherwise as in mediolateral technique (axillary tissues pulled far forward)

Alignment

— Projection: craniocaudad or mediolateral, perpendicular to the film

— Respiration suspended

Imaging Technique

Film size: 8 × 10" (18 × 24 cm)
Film speed: special mammography films
FFD: 24" (60 cm)
Bucky: yes
Focal spot: large
Exposure: 25–35 kV, automatic
— in small breasts, the photocell is moved anteriorly (close to the thorax)
— in older patients or large breasts, the photocell is moved posteriorly (away from the chest wall)

Patient Preparation
— Remove clothes from the waist up

Positioning

Craniocaudad
— Patient stands before the vertical mammography unit
— The breast is placed in the center of the cassette, height of the bucky is adjusted to position the nipple tangentially to the plane of the film
— With the hand of the side being examined, the patient grasps the handlebar on the side of the machine (the elbow is turned up to tighten the glandular tissues in the axilla)
— The patient's upper body is rotated slightly away from the machine (to completely include the outer quadrants too)
Mediolateral
— The C-arm is rotated 90°
— Patient stands with the lateral side of the breast towards the machine
— Upper body leans forward, abdomen pulled in
— Arm is flexed at the elbow, the hand grasps the handlebar
— The breast is positioned in the center, and the body rotated to the side to be examined until the nipple is tangential to the plane of the film
— The technician pulls the breast carefully forward onto the bucky tray
— The breast is now compressed (breast is pulled anteriorly, and, as compression is increased, the technician's hand slides out from under the compression paddle towards the nipple)
  Try to avoid skin folds; in the lateral projection in particular, the axillary fold should be visible without any superimposition
— Gonads shielded (small lead apron)

Contrast Examinations

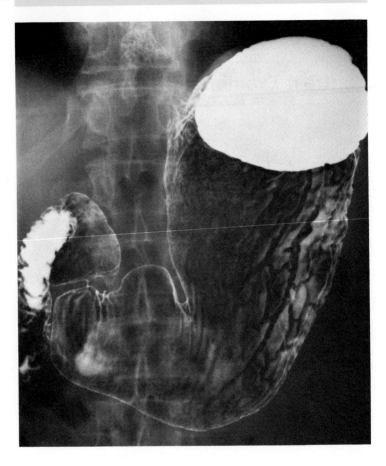

Patient Preparation
— Patient fasting; avoids nicotine

Materials and Radiographic Technique
— Cup of high-density contrast material (approx. 200 g barium sulfate/ 100 mL or oral Micropaque)
— Drinking cup for the contrast (about 150–220 mL)
— Drinking cup with about 10–15 mL water
— Bag with CO_2 granules (or 1 heaped teaspoon of effervescent powder [about 300 mL air])
— 18 gauge needle
— 2 mL syringe with 2 mL Buscopan (20 mg) (caution: glaucoma and tachycardia) or
— Insulin syringe with 15 graduations = 0.4 mg Glucagon
— Skin preparation, sponges, tourniquet
— *Film sizes:* two 8 × 10", three 10 × 12" films
— Exposure: 90–110 kV
— Starting position of the fluoro unit: upright
— All films are taken in expiration

Examining Technique
— Injection of Buscopan or Glucagon (supine)
— One swallow of contrast material (about 16–20 mL)
1st film: anterior wall/rugal relief pattern
— Prone position; 8 × 10" (18 × 24 cm), crosswise
— Have patient drink the rest of the contrast (leave enough for one swallow) in upright position
— Observe the esophagus
2nd film: fill-up views of the distended stomach (the lesser curvature is projected free, rapid examination is necessary)
— Upright position; 10 × 12" (24 × 30 cm), lengthwise
— Have patient drink the effervescent powder with water
— Turn patient on left side and tilt table horizontally
— Have patient turn from the left lateral position onto the abdomen, then turn left again over onto back
— This procedure should be repeated 3 times in order to get good contrast coating
— If the patient has difficulties turning, have him or her make rocking motions lying on the left side
— Finally, have patient turn slowly to the right side and onto the stomach, then to the left side (if the coating is poor, the procedure should be repeated)

3rd film: double-contrast view
— Supine position: 10 × 12", crosswise (or lenghtwise)
4th film: double-contrast spot films
— Have patient turn from the left side onto back; 10 × 12", crosswise,
  divided for four spot views
  1st exposure: antrum with pylorus, duodenal bulb
  2nd exposure: gastric angle and lower body region
  3rd exposure: upper body and gastric fundus with hiatal junction
  (Schatzki position), patient turned slightly to the right side, table tilted
  45° (the contrast material flows into the antrum and back to the cardia)
Check for hiatal hernia in this position:
— Have patient take a swallow of the contrast material, then tilt the table
  to lower the head
— Prone position, left side slightly elevated, have patient bear down. If
  findings are abnormal:
  4th exposure: esophageal hiatus hernia
  or
  4th exposure: gastric fundus and cardia (upright)
5th film: compression spot films
— Upright; 8 × 10", crosswise, divided into four spots, compression cone
  1st exposure: antrum
  2nd exposure: greater curvature
  3rd exposure: duodenal bulb
  4th exposure: varies, e.g., lesser curvature, duodenal bulb

Variations

First variation in examining technique
If the duodenal bulb does not unfold during the first exposure (together
with the antrum), it can be rechecked later during the series of films. Be-
tween 4th and 5th films (even with hiatal hernia) take an additional
6th film:
— 8 × 10", crosswise, divided for two views
  For example:
  1st view: fundus and cardia
  2nd view: duodenal bulb
  Then continued with the 5th film: compression views (see above)
Second variation in examining technique
Start out right away with double-contrast views:
— Materials and technique as above
— Films: two 8 × 10", two 10 × 12"

1st film: double-contrast view
— Supine position; 10 × 12", crosswise (or lengthwise)
2nd film: double-contrast spot films
— Have patient turn from the left side onto the back; 10 × 12", crosswise, divided for four spot views
  1st exposure: antrum with pylorus, duodenal bulb
  2nd exposure: gastric angle and lower body region
  3rd exposure: upper body and gastric fundus with hiatal junction (Schatzki position), patient turned slightly to the right side, table tilted 45° (the contrast material flows into the antrum and back to the cardia)
Check for hiatal hernia in this position:
— Have patient take a swallow of the contrast material, then tilt the table to lower the head
— Prone position, left side slightly elevated, have patient bear down. If findings are abnormal:
  4th exposure: esophageal hiatus hernia
  or
  4th exposure: gastric fundus and cardia (upright)
3rd film: fill-up view of the stomach (lesser curvature projected free)
Upright position; 10 × 12" (24 × 30 cm), lengthwise
4th film: compression spot films
Upright position; 8 × 10" (18 × 24 cm), crosswise, divided into four views, compression cone
  1st exposure: antrum
  2nd exposure: greater curvature
  3rd exposure: duodenal bulb
  4th exposure: varies, e.g., lesser curvature, bulb
Variation by indication
— If there is a question of gastric outlet obstruction, perforation, or foreign body, use iodinated contrast medium
— films as needed, at least one 10 × 12" survey film, in some cases 8 × 10", crosswise, divided in two

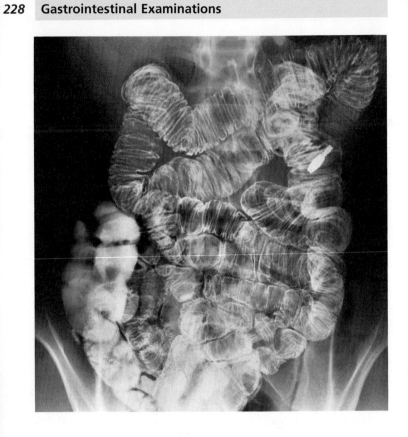

Patient Preparation

— Laxative (e.g., Dulcolax) the afternoon before the examination, liquid meal in the evening
— Fasting, nothing po the day of examination
— Patient should have a full bladder for the examination

Materials

— Plastic tube with small metal tip
— Guide wire
— Mucosal anesthetic (e.g., Xylocaine Gel) or spray for oral intubation
— Two catheter tip syringes
— Two vessels for contrast medium and methylcellulose
— Adapter for connecting syringe and tube
  or
— Pump and containers for the contrast medium and cellulose, with appropriate tubing
— Contrast and distension preparations (G. Antes method): 500 (to 900) mL diluted contrast medium (specific weight 1.2–1.3, e.g., Micropaque diluted 1:2 with water), 1500 (to 2000) mL methylcellulose (10 g dissolved in 0.2 L water heated to about 60° C and mixed well, 1800 mL cold water added and mixed once more). Instillation temperature 18° C (or body temperature)
— Films: three 10 × 12" (24 × 30 cm), two 14 × 17" (35 × 35)
— Exposure: 110–130 kV

Examining Technique

— Preliminary fluoroscopic check (for residual contrast, free air, bowel-gas pattern)
— After local anesthesia of the nasopharynx, the tube, with stiff guide wire, is inserted through the nose, with the patient erect
— The tube is then advanced, and the patient is put into a horizontal position (first on the right side to pass through the pylorus, then on the left side for passage through the duodenal loop, tip of the tube flexible)
— Distal portion of the tube is advanced beyond the ligament of Treitz (to prevent reflux)
— Contrast instillation, first under fluoro, of about 300 mL at a flow rate of 80 mL/min

1st film: single contrast view of the jejunum
— 10 × 12" (24 × 30 cm), crosswise or lengthwise
— Immediate and quick instillation of methylcellulose at a flow rate of about 100–200 mL/min; total volume mostly 500–1500 mL, depending on the length of the intestine

2nd–3rd film: jejunum and ileum, double contrast views, cecum
— 24 × 30 cm, divided as necessary for good demonstration, compression spots if needed

4th–5th film: jejunum and ileum, double-contrast views (survey films, depending on findings; either oblique or in prone and supine positions) — 14 × 17" (35 × 35 cm)

Followed By
— Tube removal

Variations
Variation in examining technique – J. Desaga Method

Patient Preparation
— Oral administration of three doses of 200 mg acetylcysteine 2 days before the examination
  Otherwise as described above

Materials
— Contrast medium: 2 g Guarine (e.g., HP-7000 = 2/1 measuring spoons mixed with 3 mL glycerin, and added to a 1 : 1 barium sulfate–water suspension, or, e.g., 200 mL Micropaque and 200 mL tap water); ready for use after 4 hrs
— Distension solution: 15 g Guarine (e.g., HP-7000 = 5/1 measuring spoons) mixed with 20 mL glycerin and added to 3000 mL tap water; let stand and expand for 4 hrs, then it is ready for use and keeps in the refrigerator for 24 hrs
— Heat to 98.6° F (37 °C) before use
— Have Glucagon ready
— Tubes, syringes, or pump, as above
Examination technique as above
(The distension medium is instilled at the rate of 100–120 mL/min)
Variation in radiographic technique
Camera instead of fluoroscopic spots on 10 × 12" film

Tips & Tricks
When in doubt, use less contrast and more methylcellulose. If this results in poor contrast visualization of the proximal jejunum because of too much dilution, 50–100 mL barium can be added in between the methylcellulose injections.

Patient Preparation
— Two days before the examination, begin dietary and laxative (e.g., X-Prep, Dulcolax) preparations as per instruction

Materials and Radiographic Technique
— Contrast medium (about 50 g barium sulfate/100 mL approx. 1–1.5 L, warmed up)
— Disposable enema bag with hose, enema tip (olive), and Y-connection with rubber ball for air insufflation (e.g., pneumocolon)
— Contrast pump with connections and colon tube (additional pressure gauge and connections)
— Films: four 10 × 12" (24 × 30 cm), two 14 × 17" (35 × 35 cm)
— Exposure: 90–110 kV
— Starting position of the fluoro unit: horizontal

Examining Technique
— Preliminary fluoroscopic check (for residual contrast, calcifications, free air?)
— Brief rectal examination (stenosis, tumor; blood or feces on glove?)
— Insert rectal tip
— Patient lies on the left side
— Instillation of the contrast medium under fluoroscopic control and under increased pressure if necessary (e.g., contrast pump)
— Retrograde flow of the contrast medium past the splenic flexure into the beginning or distal portion of the transverse colon
— The contrast is then advanced further just beyond the right flexure by turning the patient on the right side or by air insufflation
— Have the patient get up and evacuate the contrast material (either into the enema bag, or patient is sent to the toilet)
— Next, air insufflation with the patient lying on the left side (pump with controlled pressure if needed), under fluoroscopic control until the bowel segments of interest are distended
1st film: sigmoid rotated free of superimposed bowel loops
— Positioning under fluoroscopy (supine position, either left or right side slightly turned up)
— 10 × 12" (24 × 30 cm), crosswise, undivided

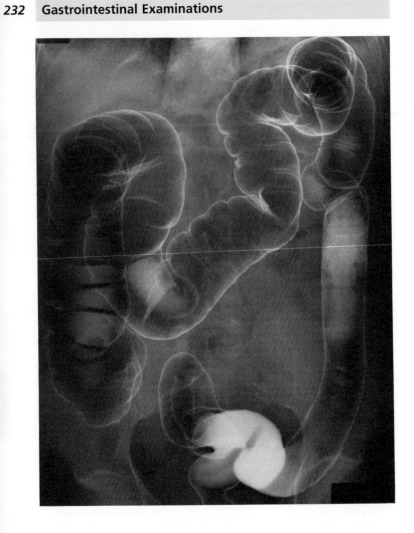

2nd film:
— 10 × 12" (24 × 30 cm), crosswise, divided in two
1st exposure: double-contrast view of the lateral rectum (shows the anterior margin of the sacrum, femoral heads are superimposed on each other), left lateral position
2nd exposure: double-contrast view of the AP rectum, supine position (or prone, with head lowered)
3rd film: AP view of the transverse colon (cecum may also be clearly projected)
— Supine position
— 14 × 17" (35 × 35 cm), undivided
4th film: left colonic (splenic) flexure
— Positioned fluoroscopically, erect, usually LAO
— 10 × 12", lengthwise, undivided
5th film: right colonic (hepatic) flexure
— Positioned fluoroscopically, erect, usually RAO
— 10 × 12", lengthwise, undivided
6th film: survey film
— Erect AP
— 14 × 17" (35 × 35 cm), undivided

Variations

Variation in examining technique: hypotonic study of the colon
Materials (in addition to the above)
— 18 gauge needle
— 2 mL syringe with 2 mL Buscopan (20 mg) (caution: glaucoma and tachycardia)
   or
— Insulin syringe with 15 graduations = 0.4 mg Glucagon
— Skin preparation, sponges, tourniquet
— Injection of Buscopan (20 mg) (or glucagon) prior to the instillation (or when needed)
Variation in radiographic technique: bucky table method (Welin technique)
Films: six 10 × 12" five 14 × 17" (30 × 40 cm)
Other materials and technique as above
1st film: double-contrast view of the rectum, PA
— Prone position
— 10 × 12" (24 × 30 cm), undivided

4th film: rectum, lateral projcetion
— Left lateral position
— 10 × 12" (24 × 30 cm), lengthwise, undivided
5th and 6th films: supine films of the abdomen, right and left oblique views
— Supine position, 30°–45° rotation, centered at the umbilicus
— 14 × 17" (30 × 40 cm), undivided
7th film: recumbent film of the abdomen, horizontal projection
— Left lateral position, centered at the umbilicus
— 14 × 17" (30 × 40 cm), undivided
8th film: recumbent film of the abdomen, horizontal projection
— Right lateral position, centered at the umbilicus
— 14 × 17" (30 × 40 cm), undivided
9th film: erect film of the abdomen
— Centered at the umbilicus
— 14 × 17" (30 × 40 cm), undivided
10th film: erect film of the abdomen (for the right colonic flexure)
— 45° RAO, centered 2 FB above the umbilicus, right upper abdomen
— 14 × 17" (30 × 40 cm), undivided
11th film: erect film of the abdomen (for the left colonic flexure)
— 45° LAO, centered 4 FB above the umbilicus, left upper abdomen
— 14 × 17" (30 × 40 cm), undivided

Complications and What-to-Do

— Rectum perforation: Special caution at the beginning of the contrast- and air-instillation
— Pains during the insufflation of air: may be due to overdistension of a bowel segment. Change the patient's position (turn the more proximal, undistended bowel loop upward)
— If the bowel loops, don't dilate: inject Buscopan (see *Variations*)

Patient Preparation
— Nothing p.o. (per os) or orally 3 hrs prior to the examination
— Laxatives and bowel cleansing the day before
— Creatinine less than 3 mg/dL (with larger doses of contrast medium up to 6 mg/dL)

Materials and Radiographic Technique
— Contrast medium (dosage: adults 1 mL/kg body weight; children up to 1 yr, 3 mL/kg body weight, [20 mL maximum, 12 mL minimum dose]; up to 2 yrs, 2.5 mL/kg body weight [20 mL maximum dose]; up to 3 yrs, 1.5 mL/kg body weight [25 mL maximum dose]; mostly 60%)
— Butterfly or indwelling catheter (21 or 18 gauge)
Films: two 14 × 17" (under ideal conditions)
Film speed: 400
FFD: 40" (115 cm)
Focal spot: large
Exposure: 70–75 kV, automatic, all cells

Examining Technique
1st film: 14 × 17" (35 × 43 cm), lengthwise, undivided
— Preliminary film
— Supine position, lower film edge = upper border of the pubic symphysis
— Additional oblique or preliminary tomographic view
— Injection of the contrast medium
2nd film: 14 × 17" (35 × 43 cm), lengthwise, undivided
— 14 min after the injection
— Supine position, lower film edge = upper border of the pubic symphysis
— Additional views as needed
Zonography
— 10 × 12" (24 × 30 cm), undivided
— Linear blurring, 8° exposure angle
— Depth of cuts about 8–9 cm, exposure time about 2 seconds
— Supine position, centering over the kidney region (upper cassette border at about the level of the xiphoid process)
If *tomographic views* are required
— Three 10 × 12", lengthwise, undivided
— Linear blurring, 30° amplitude
— Tomographic cuts at 1 cm intervals
— Centering over the kidneys
— Tomographic cuts at 9, 10, 11 cm (normal patients)

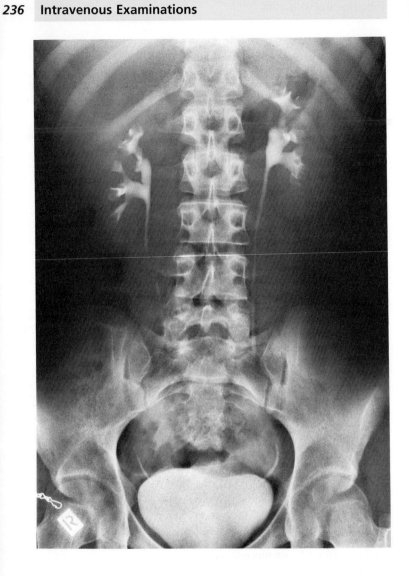

Lateral oblique views if needed
Compression films (for better filling of the renal pelves)
(Caution with compression if there is obstruction of urinary drainage or infection)
— Either application of compression belt or patient in prone position, film taken after 15 minutes
Either
— 10 × 12" (24 × 30 cm), crosswise, undivided
— Supine position, centering over the kidneys
or
— 14 × 17" (43 × 35 cm), lengthwise, undivided
— Supine position (remove compression belt)
— Lower film edge = upper border of the symphysis
Bladder films
1st film: full bladder
— 10 × 12" (24 × 30 cm), lengthwise, undivided
— Lower film edge = 2 cm below upper border of the symphysis
2nd film: bladder post voiding
— 8 × 10" (18 × 24 cm), crosswise, undivided
— Lower film edge = 2 cm below upper border of the symphysis
All films are taken in expiration and suspended respiration
Delayed films for follow-up (e.g., nonfunctioning kidney, obstruction): 30 min, 1, 2, 12, 24 hrs post injection

Variations
(as part of excretory function studies)
— Erect urogram in lateral projection, at rest, and attempting to strain and bear down
— Early urogram in AP supine position in case of suspected renal artery stenosis
— Breathing urogram to evaluate inflammatory fixation of the kidney in AP projection with long exposure time and low mA
— Oblique views for question of ureteral calculus: opposite side turned up 45° (if calculus is suspected behind the bladder, same side obliqued 45°)

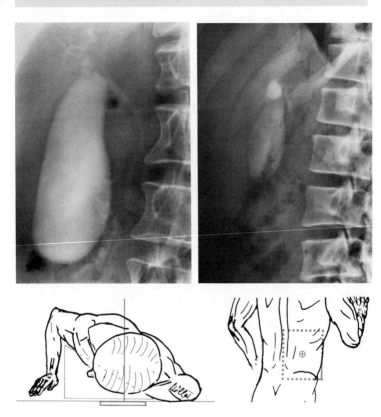

Variations

Variation of the examination technique: combining "i.v. gallbladder" and "oral gallbladder" examinations

— Scout film (see above) and administration of the oral cholegraphic contrast medium the day before
— Injection of the i.v. contrast medium on the day of examination (the continued as above)

Tips & Tricks

— Too rapid contrast injection can cause nausea (because of hepatocellular passage limits)
— If the patient has had a previous cholecystectomy, the examination is terminated after the 3rd film if there is good contrast visualization of the bile ducts

Patient Preparation
— Patient fasting for 12 hrs
— Bilirubin (less than 5 mg/dL)
— Scout film (see below)

Materials
20 mg cholegraphic contrast medium (as a short infusion in about 10–15 min)
— Intracath or butterfly needle (21 or 18 gauge)
— Fatty meal
— Films: five 10 × 12" (24 × 30 cm)

Examining Technique
1st film: preliminary scout film
— Contrast unfusion (50 mL in 30 min or contrast injection 30 mL in 50 min)
2nd film: (optional) 15 min after injection
3rd film: 30 min after injection
— additional views in 30 to 60 minutes until the gallbladder is homogeneously opacified
Tomography of the bile ducts
— Three 10 × 12", lengthwise, undivided
— Linear blurring, 8° exposure angle
— Tomographic cuts at 1 cm intervals
— Cuts at 7, 8, 9 cm depth (normal patients)
— Otherwise, same as plain films of the gallbladder
4th film:
— 10 × 12", crosswise, divided in two (fluoroscopy)
— compression cone in place
   1st exposure: upright fluoroscopic positioning and compression to separate and project the gallbladder and bile ducts
   2nd exposure; supine, fluoroscopic positioning and compression to free the projection of the gallbladder
— Oral administration of the fatty meal (caution: danger of colic if concretions are present)
5th film: 30 min after the fatty meal
6th film:
— 10 × 12", crosswise, divided in two (fluoroscopy)
— compression cone in place
   1st exposure: upright fluoroscopic positioning and compression to separate and project the gallbladder and bile ducts
   2nd exposure: supine, fluoroscopic positioning and compression to free the projection of the gallbladder

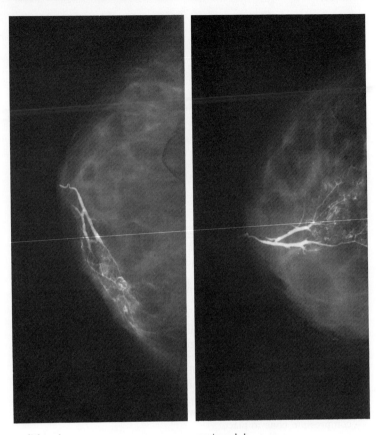

mediolateral   craniocaudad

Patient Preparation
— Mammography in two planes

Materials (sterile)
— Plastic tube with attached blunt cannula with end hole (e.g., galactography set) or dilators sizes 7, 8 and blunt cannulas sizes 7, 8
— 2 mL syringe with contrast medium (50%)
— Spray dressing
— Sterile towels, sponges, gloves
— Skin disinfectant

Examining Technique
— After cleaning the nipple, controlled compression of the breast until the opening of the secreting mammary duct becomes moist
— Smear of mamillary secretion for cytological examination
— Dilatation of the duct, if necessary
— Insertion of the blunt cannula
— Lifting and compression of the nipple
— Injection of 0.5–2 mL contrast medium (no air!)
— Watch for patient's sensations of discomfort (feelings of tenseness, drawing pains)
— After removal of the cannula, closure of the mammary duct by compression (and spray dressing if necessary)

Radiographs
Mammography in two planes with moderate compression to prevent leaking of the contrast medium

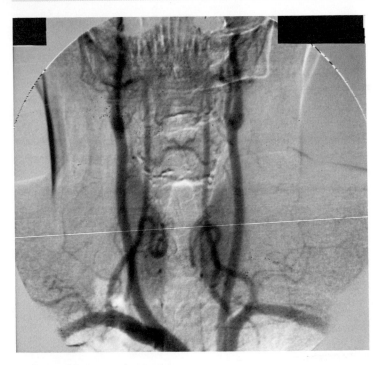

Radiographic Protocol

— At least two films/sec
— After breathing instructions, contrast medium is injected, breath is held in midrespiration
— Masks are prepared at the same time
— Wait for the end of the venous phase (series takes about 12 sec, prolonged to 20 sec if there is arterial occlusion, e.g., subclavian steal syndrome)
— Series is terminated

1st series
— Survey film of the aortic arch (30°–45° LAO, 10°–20° craniocaudad tube angulation for origin of the great vessels)

2nd series
— Neck LAO, head turned left (with electronic image magnification

3rd series
— Neck RAO, head turned right (with electronic image magnification)

4th series
— Neck AP, 30°–40° craniocaudad tube angulation (with electronic magnification, cervicocranial vascular junction)

Patient Preparation
— Nothing p.o. for at least 3 hrs
— Explanation of the procedure, obtain consent

Equipment and Materials
DSA table (peripheral venous)
— Two large syringes (20 or 30 mL) with NaCl
— 2 mL syringe with 21 gauge needle for local anesthesia
— Sponges
— Skin disinfectant (Betadine)
— Tourniquet
— Sterile bandages
Catheters
— Intracath or butterfly needles 14 and 16 gauge
— High-pressure two-way stopcock
— High-pressure connection tube, with clamps to attach to the table

Positioning
— Supine

Technical Preparations
— Fill the injection syringe

Puncture
— After local anesthesia, needle puncture of the median cubital vein
— Connecting tube attached (make sure there is no air in the tubing)
— Test injection of saline under rapid flow
— Connection to the injector (connecting tube fastened and high-pressure two-way stopcock)
— Raise the arm above the head to straighten the inflow tract

Injection Parameters
— About 50 mL nonionic contrast medium
— Injection speed:
  about 14–16 mL/sec with 16 gauge needle
  about 18–22 mL/sec with 14 gauge needle

Postoperative Care
— Check for reaction to the contrast medium
— Pressure dressing

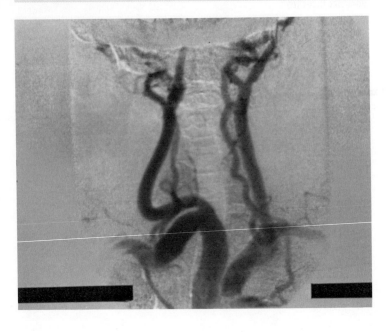

Patient Preparation
— Nothing p.o. for at least 3 hrs
— Clotting tests (Quick Test, PT, PTT), creatinine
— Chest X-ray
— Explanation of the procedure, obtain consent

Equipment and Materials
DSA table (central venous, sterile)
— Basin with NaCl and heparin (200 IU/10 mL)
— Two large syringes (20 or 30 mL) for NaCl
— One large syringe (20–30 mL, Luer–Lock) for the contrast medium
— 10 mL syringe with 21 and 23 gauge needles for local anesthesia
— Puncture needle (e.g., 18 gauge for 0.38' or 19 gauge for 0.35' guide wire)
— Scalpel
— High-pressure two-way stopcock
— Sterile sponges (10 small, 10 large)
— Sterile towels, gloves
— Contrast medium, local anesthetic
— Skin disinfectant (e.g., Betadine)
— Disposable razor for femoral vein
Catheters
— 5 French pigtail catheter, length 65 cm (or straight catheter with side holes, 5 French, length 65 cm)
— Puncture needle (e.g., 18 gauge for 0.38' or 19 gauge for 0.35' guide wire)
— Or 4 French pigtail catheter (attention to flow and guide-wire diameter)

Positioning
— Supine position

Technical Preparations
— Syringe filled for injection, free of air

Puncture
— Femoral or median cubital vein punctured after local anesthesia and skin incision
— The catheter is advanced along the inserted guide wire into the superior vena cava just above the right atrium
— Trial injection to check position
— Connection to the injector (after the air is out)

(continued from p. 247)

Injection Parameters
— About 30–50 mL nonionic contrast medium
— Injection speed: 15–20 mL/sec.

Radiographic Protocol
— At least two films/sec
— After breathing instructions, injection of the contrast medium, respiration suspended in expiration
— At the same time, a mask is prepared
— Wait for the venous phase (series takes about 12 sec, as long as 20 sec if there is arterial occlusion (e.g., subclavian steal syndrome)
— Terminate the series

1st series
— Survey films of the aortic arch (30°–45° LAO, 10°–20° craniocaudad tube angulation for origin of the great vessels)

2nd series
— Neck LAO, head turned left (with electronic image magnification)

3rd series
— Neck RAO, head turned right (with electronic image magnification)

4th series
— Neck AP, 30°–40° craniocaudad tube angulation (with electronic image magnification, cervicocranial vascular junction)

Postoperative Care
— Check for reaction to the contrast medium
— About 5 min compression (of the femoral vein)
— Pressure dressing applied to the puncture site
— Recheck about 1/2 hr before discharge

Patient Preparation
— Nothing p.o. for 3 hrs
— Clotting tests (Quick Test, PTT, thrombocytes)
— Chest X-ray in two projections
— Explanation of the procedure, obtain consent

Equipment and Materials
Angio table (sterile)
— Basin with NaCl and heparin (200 IU/100 mL)
— Two large syringes (20 or 30 mL)
— One large contrast syringe (Luer–Lock, 20 mL)
— 10 mL syringe with 21 and 23 gauge needles for local anesthesia
— Sponges (10 small, 10 large)
— Scalpel
— Puncture needle (e.g., 18 gauge for 0.38' or 19 gauge for 0.35' guide wire)
— High-pressure two-way stopcock
— Sterile towels
— Sterile coat, gloves
— Disposable razor
— Skin disinfectant (e. g., Betadine)
— Contrast medium, local anesthetic
Catheters
— 5 French pigtail catheter (100 cm)
— J-guide with soft tip (e.g., 0.38' or 0.35' 120–150 cm length)

Positioning

— Supine position
— Shaving of the inguinal areas
— Skin disinfection
— Cover with sterile towels

Technical Preparations
— Syringe filled for injection, free of air

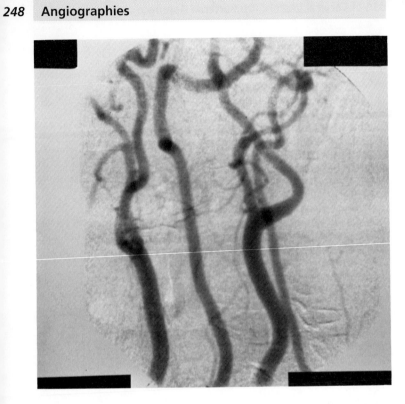

Puncture (Seldinger Technique)
— Femoral artery punctured after local anesthesia (pulsating jet of blood)
— Insertion of the J-guide
— Puncture needle is removed
— Catheter is inserted and advanced forward along the guide
— The guide is then removed
— Catheter placed at the origin of the ascending aorta (about 2 cm distal to the aortic valve)
— Preliminary aspiration of blood, saline injection (free runoff), test dose of contrast to check position
— Connection to the injector

Injection Parameters
— 20 mL non-ionic contrast medium (350–370 mg iodine/mL)
— Injection speed 10 mL/sec
— No injection delay

Radiographic Protocol
— Four films/sec
— Injection after masks have been prepared
— Respiration suspended in expiration
1st series
— Survey films of the aortic arch (30°–45° LAO; tip: catheter turned up under fluoroscopy)
— 10°–20° craniocaudad tube angulation
2nd series
— Supine position, neck LAO (magnifying technique)
— Head turned left (about 30°–40° LAO)
3rd series
— Supine position, neck RAO (magnifying technique)
— Head turned right (about 30°–45° RAO)
4th series (optional)
— Supine position, neck AP (magnifying technique)
— 30° craniocaudad tube angulation

Postoperative Care
— Check for reaction to the contrast medium
— Compression of the puncture site for about 10 min
— Pressure dressing
— Bed rest (12–24 hrs)

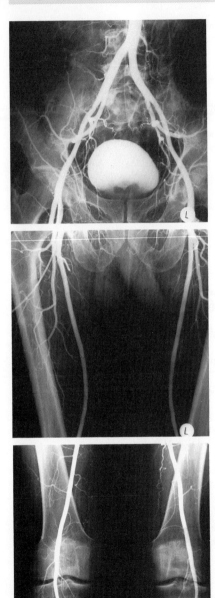

Patient Preparation
— Nothing p.o. for 3–6 hrs
— Clotting tests (e.g., Quick test greater than 50%, PT, PTT, thrombocytes)
— Creatinine
— Explanation of the procedure, obtain consent

Equipment, Materials, and Radiographic Technique
Angio table (sterile)
— Basin with NaCl and heparin (200 IU/100 mL)
— Two large syringes (20 or 30 mL) for NaCl
— One large contrast syringe (Luer–Lock, 20 mL)
— 10 mL syringe with 21 and 23 gauge needles for local anesthesia
— Sponges (10 small, 10 large)
— Scalpel
— Puncture needle (e.g., 19 gauge for 0.35' guide wire)
— Two-way stopcock
— Sterile towels
— Sterile coat, gloves
— Skin disinfectant, contrast medium, local anesthetic
— Disposable razor
— Films: load 10 cassette films
— Tube settings: about 66 kV (64 mAs [trial], negative step-down: 5, 15, 20, 25 kV)
Catheters
— 5 French pigtail catheter (65 cm)
— J-guide with soft tip (e-g., 0.35', 120–150 cm long)

Positioning

— Supine position
— Shaving of the inguinal areas
— Skin disinfection
— Cover with sterile towels

Technical Preparations
— Take a scout film (central ray about 7 cm above the umbilicus to include the renal vessels, or 7 cm below umbilicus without renal vessels)
— Syringe filled for injection

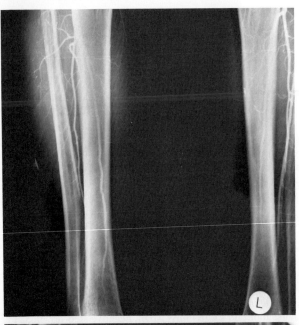

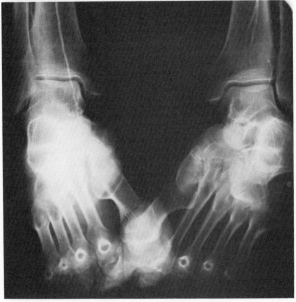

Puncture (Seldinger Technique)
— Femoral artery punctured after local anesthesia (pulsating jet of blood)
— Insertion of the J-guide
— The puncture needle is withdrawn, a dilator may be put in place
— Catheter, with open stopcock, is inserted and advanced forward along the guide
— The guide is removed, catheter flushed with NaCl, stopcock closed
— Catheter placed approx. 2 cm above the bifurcation, at about the level of L4 or at the renal artery level at L1–L2
— Test aspiration of blood, injection of NaCl (free runoff?)
— Catheter position checked with a test dose of the contrast medium
— Connection to the injector

Injection Parameters
— About 80 mL of non-ionic contrast medium
— Injection speed and delay depending on the vascular situation or the flow-test injection, or on the walking distance
— Walking distance more than 200 m: flow = 11 mL/sec, 3 sec delay
— Walking distance about 100 m: flow 10 mL/sec, 5 sec delay
— Walking distance 20–50 m: flow 8 mL/sec, 7–8 sec delay

Radiographic Protocol
— 4 table shifts = 5 filming stations
— At each station, one fim/sec twice
— Legs slightly rotated internally (with genu varum knee supported to compensate)
— Abdominal and pelvic levels in expiratory suspended respiration

Postoperative Care
— Check for reaction to the contrast medium
— 10 min compression of the puncture site
— Pressure dressing
— At least 24 hrs bed rest

Tips & Tricks
For patients less than $5^{1}/_{2}$ ft tall, only 3 table shifts = 4 filming stations = 8 cassette films are needed.

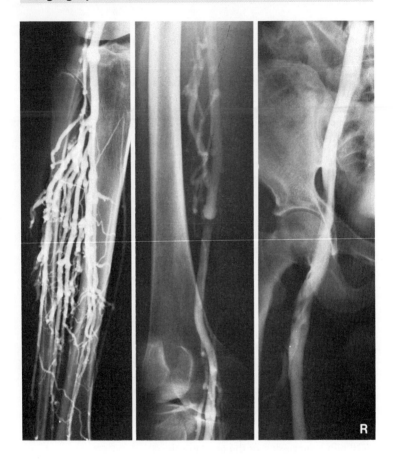

Patient Preparation
— Nothing p.o. for 3 hrs

Materials
— Butterfly needle (19–21 gauge) or intracath in case of thrombolytic therapy
— One 20 mL syringe with 0.9% saline
— Three 20 mL (or one 50 mL) syringes for contrast medium
— Tourniquet for application above the ankle
— A 2nd tourniquet for application around the distal thigh
— Sponges, Band-Aids, skin disinfectant
— Contrast medium
— Restraining belt
— Measuring rod
— Films: two 11 × 14", and two 10 × 12" held ready

Examining Technique
— Application of a tourniquet above the ankle, puncture of a superficial vein in the dorsum of the foot with a butterfly needle after the air has been let out
— Puncture as distal as possible (mostly dorsal vein of the great toe)
— About 45° table tilt with the patient supine
— So-called "hanging position" with handles for support, or patient stands on one leg on a wooden block
— Attach measuring rod
— Manual injection of the contrast medium (40–60 mL)

1st film: 11 × 14", divided in three

1st exposure: lower leg in 30° internal rotation

2nd exposure: lower leg lateral (in maximal external rotation)

3rd exposure: knee region, including distal and midthigh (lateral, have patient strain: small saphenous vein)

— Ask patient to continue to strain, in order to get good filling for the runoff phase = 4th exposure
— Patient is put into horizontal position under fluoroscopy, the leg is elevated, calf compressed (caution: possible thrombosis)

2nd film: 11 × 14", divided in three

4th exposure: middle and upper thigh (have patient strain)

If the valves of the great saphenous vein are competent, continue with

5th exposure: inguinal and iliac region

6th exposure: drainage into the inferior vena cava or delayed film of the lower leg in internal rotation

Postoperative Care
— Elevate and massage the leg
— Remove the needle, apply dressing, have patient walk up stairs
— Wrap the legs of bedridden patients

Variations
Variation in examining technique
In case of insufficiency of the great saphenous vein, the sequence of the 2nd film is changed:
4th exposure: proximal thigh and inguinal region (demonstrating the drainage into the external and common iliac veins, and insufficiency of the valve
5th exposure: proximal and midportions of the insufficient great saphenous vein
6th exposure: distal insufficiency point of the great saphenous vein

Tips & Tricks
— If not all veins of the lower leg fill right at the beginning, change the exposure sequence of the
1st film: 11 × 14", divided in three
1st exposure: lateral knee and distal thigh
2nd exposure: lateral lower leg
3rd exposure: lower leg in 30° internal rotation
— If filling is still inadequate, squeeze the contrast material manually from the forefoot
— If filling is still incomplete, 2nd injection after putting a 2nd tourniquet around the distal thigh

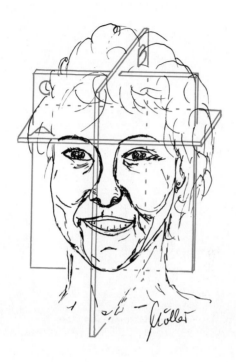

A = axial (horizontal) plane
B = sagittal plane
C = coronal (frontal) plane

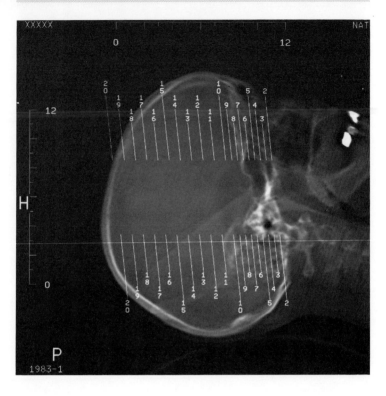

Patient Preparation
— Nothing p.o. for 3 hrs before the examination (contrast injection)

Positioning
— Supine
— Arms along the sides of the body
— Head immobilized in the head holder

Parameters
— Scan range starting at base of the skull; ending at vertex of the skull
— Respiration: shallow breathing
Unit controls
— Lateral scout view
— Gantry (radiation detector system) tilt: 0° (parallel to canthomeatal line)
— Slice thickness and slice spacing:
   4 mm from skull base to tentorial rim
   8 mm from tentorial rim to vertex
Window algorithm
— Soft-tissue window:
   Posterior fossa:
   window level (WL) 40–60 HU
   window width (WW) 120 HU
   Rest of the neurocranium:
   WL 35–50 HU
   WW 70–100 HU

Variation
— If there are pathological findings or questions of tumor or metastases: i.v. injection of 50 mL nonionic contrast medium (Omnipaque 300) before the examination
— If there is a possibility of a fracture: bone-window level (WL) 300–600 HU, width (WW) 1000–2000 HU
— In cases of occipital or petrous bone fractures: slice thickness 2 mm, slice spacing 2 mm, high resolution (HRCT) technique (if available), bone window

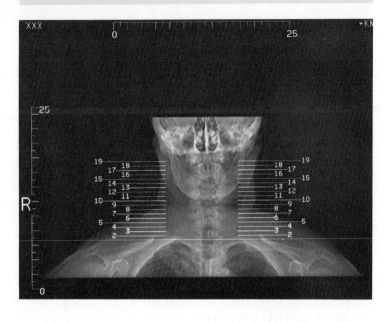

Patient Preparation
— Nothing p.o. for 3 hrs before the examination (contrast injection)

Contrast Medium
— Infusion of 100–150 mL nonionic contrast medium (Omnipaque 300)

Positioning
— Supine
— Arms along the sides of the body
— Immobilization of the head

Parameters
— Scan range
  starting at floor of the mouth;
  ending at supraclavicular fossa
— Respiration: suspended in expiration, no swallowing
Unit controls
— Topogram (scanogram): AP, when necessary
— Gantry tilt: 0°
— Slice thickness: 4 mm
— Slice spacing: 6 mm
— Prescan magnified scout view: floor of the mouth or neck encompassing the display field of view
Window algorithm
— Soft-tissue window:
  WL 40–60 HU
  WW 300 HU

Variation
— Bolus injection of 100 mL contrast medium for spiral CT or "dynamic scan"

Tips & Tricks
Inject 20 mL contrast medium as an i.v. bolus directly before the examination, followed by a fast infusion of contrast.

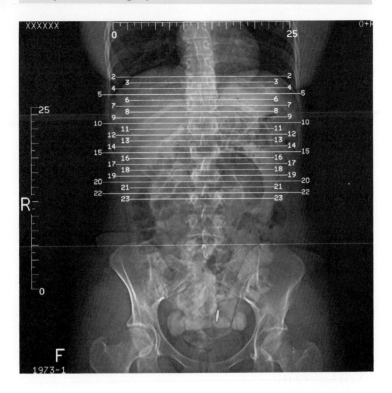

Patient Preparation
— Nothing p.o. for 3 hrs before the examination (contrast injection)
— Chest X-ray in two projections

Positioning
— Supine
— Arms folded behind the head

Parameters
— Scan range starting
   at pulmonary apex;
   ending at marginal sinus (inferior aspect of the CPA)
— Respiration: suspended in inspiration
Unit controls
— AP scout view
— Gantry tilt: 0°
— Slice thickness: 8–10 mm
— Slice spacing: 8–10 mm
Window algorithm
— Soft-tissue window:
   WL 40–60 HU
   WW 200–500 HU
— Lung window:
   WL –s600 to –800 HU
   WW 1000–2000 HU

Variation
If there are pathological findings, especially in the hilar region:
— Bolus injection (with injector) of 100 mL nonionic contrast medium
   (Omnipaque 300) targeted to the lesion
— Change slice thickness to 4 mm or 2mm
— Possibly HRCT technique for certain regions
— For CT of the chest in children, slice thickness may be reduced to
   5 mm

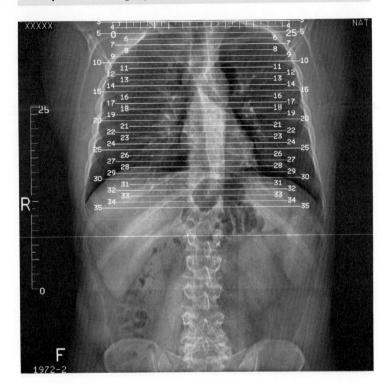

Patient Preparation
— Nothing p.o. for 3 hrs before the examination

Contrast Media
— About $1/2$–1 hr before the examination, 500 mL of iodinated CT contrast material in a 3% dilution are given orally if necessary (caution: hyperthyroidism, allergy), or Micropaque CT
— The last 100 mL are given immediately before the examination, with regard to the diagnostic problem (pancreas, for instance)
— If more contrast is needed, i.v. injection of nonionic contrast medium (100 mL Omnipaque 300)
— Injection of Buscopan (glucagon) to suppress intestinal motility

Positioning
— Supine
— Arms folded behind the head

Parameters
— Scan range
  starting at dome of the diaphragm;
  ending, depending on the problem, at least at lower kidney pole
— Respiration: suspended in expiration
Unit controls
— AP scout view
— Gantry tilt: 0°
— Slice thickness: 8–10 mm
— Slice spacing: 8–10 mm
Window algorithm
— Soft-tissue window:
  WL 40–60 HU
  WW 200–500 HU

Tips & Tricks
— Patient turned briefly on the right side (for contrast filling of the duodenum)
— Scanning with patient on the right side if there are questionable findings in the pancreas
— For demonstrating pancreatic abnormalities, choose 4 mm slice thickness and spacing

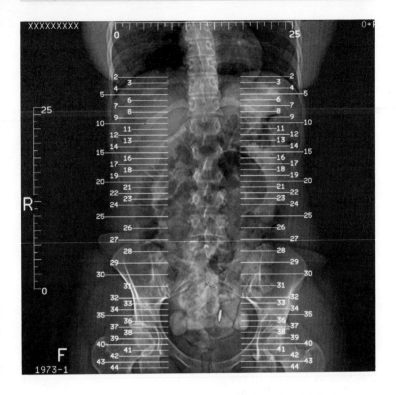

Patient Preparation
— Nothing p.o. for 3 hrs before the examination (contrast injection)

Contrast Media
Patient given 1000 mL oral contrast medium (e.g., Micropaque CT or iodinated contrast medium in 3% dilution) in fractionated doses from 1½ hrs until shortly before the beginning of the examination (caution: hyperthyroidism, allergy)
— Shortly before the examination, patient takes a few more swallows of the contrast medium
— A vaginal tampon may be inserted, if indicated
— Rectal instillation of about 500–1000 mL of suitable contrast material
— Injection of Buscopan (glucagon) to suppress intestinal motility
— Bolus injection of 100 mL nonionic contrast medium (Omnipaque 300)

Positioning
— Supine
— Arms folded behind the head

Parameters
— Scan range
   starting at dome of the diaphragm;
   ending at the lower ischial border
— Respiration: suspended in expiration
Unit controls
— AP scout view if indicated
— Gantry tilt: 0°
— Slice thickness: 8–10 mm
— Slice spacing:
   8–10 mm from the dome of the diaphragm to the lower border of the kidney and lesser pelvis, 16–20 mm for the rest of the abdomen
Window algorithm
— Soft-tissue window:
   WL 40–50 HU
   WW 200–500 HU

Tips & Tricks
Take delayed films if there is poor contrast visualization of the bowel, for instance, or after i.v. contrast injection shows suspicious renal or urinary bladder findings

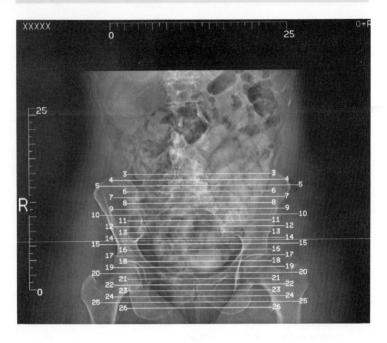

Patient Preparation
— Nothing p.o. for 3 hrs before the examination (contrast injection)
— Patient should not void before the examination (the study is done with full bladder)

Contrast Media
— About 1¹/₂–2 hrs before the examination, patient is given 1000 mL oral CT contrast (e.g., iodinated contrast medium in 3% dilution: caution: hyperthyroidism, allergy), or Micropaque CT
— A vaginal tampon may be inserted, if indicated
— Rectal instillation of warmed, suitable contrast material (about 500 mL, or 250 mL as a one-time enema)
— Injection of Buscopan (Glucagon) to suppress intestinal motility
— Bolus injection of 100 mL nonionic contrast medium (Omnipaque 300)

Positioning
— Supine
— Arms folded behind the head or on the chest

Parameters
— Scan range
  starting at the iliac crest,
  ending at the lower ischial border
— Respiration: suspended in expiration or shallow breathing
Unit controls
— AP scout view
— Gantry tilt: 0°
— Slice thickness:
  8–10 mm, 2–5 mm through areas of special concern (e.g., prostatic or bladder tumor)
— Slice spacing:
  8–10 mm, less through areas of special concern (see thickness)
Window algorithm
— Soft-tissue window:
  WL 40–60 HU
  WW 200–500 HU

Tips & Tricks
Take delayed films 20–30 min after contrast injection, with full bladder and thin-slice technique, if there are questionable bladder or prostate findings.

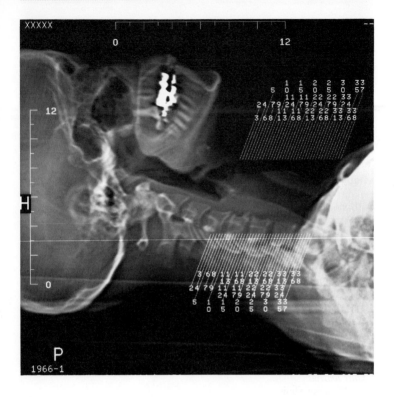

Patient Preparation
— Cervical spine films in two projections
— Neurological evaluation

Positioning
— Supine
— Arms along the sides of the body
— Have shoulders pulled down (with assistance, e.g., sling or band tied around the feet, etc.)

Parameters
— Scan range
    starting—as clinicall indicated;
    ending—as clinically indicated
— Respiration: suspended, no swallowing
Unit controls
— Lateral scout view
— Gantry tilt:
    parallel to the intervertebral disc, the angle is maintained and followed through (for better reconstruction)
— Slice thickness: 2–4 mm
— Slice spacing: 2–4 mm
Window algorithm
— Soft-tissue window:
    WL 30–40 HU
    WW 200–300 HU
— If bone window:
    WL 200–500 HU
    WW 1000–1800 HU

Variations
CT myelography (see p. 275, CT scan of the lumbar spine)

Tips & Tricks
— Get a scout view for all scans
— Sagittal reconstruction of abnormal scans (bone and soft-tissue window algorithms)
— Identify and label the vertebral levels (C4, C5) or their corresponding intervertebral spaces (C4/C5)

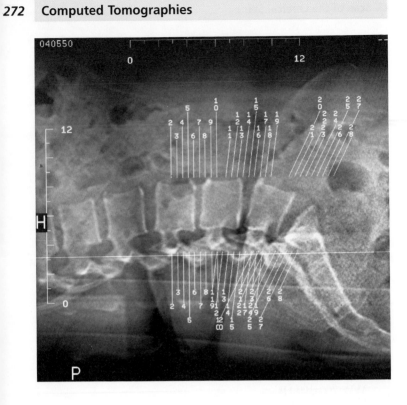

Patient Preparation
— Lumbar and thoracic spine in two projections
— Neurological evaluation

Positioning
— Supine
— Arms folded behind the head or on the chest
— Straighten the lumbar lordosis for CT with a knee roll or by putting a wedge pillow under the pelvis

---

Parameters
— Scan range
    starting—as clinically indicated;
    ending—as clinically indicated
— Respiration: shallow breathing
Unit controls
— Lateral scout view
— Gantry tilt: parallel to the intervetebral disc or to the vertebral plate
— Slice thickness: 2–4 mm
— Slice spacing: 4 mm
Window algorithm
— Soft-tissue window:
    WL 30–40 HU
    WW 200–300 HU
— If bone window:
    WL 300–500 HU
    WW 1000–1800 HU

Variation: CT Myelography

Materials (sterile)
— Spinal needle (20 gauge) or special Myelography needle
— 10 mL syringe with 10 mL nonionic contrast medium (e.g., Omnipaque 180)
— Spinal ("eye"-) drape, gloves, sponges
— Skin disinfectant (Betadine spray)
— Contrast medium (for additional injection)
— Sterile test tubes (for spinal-fluid examination)
— Sponge wedge
Positioning
— Patient lies on side, knees drawn up
— Neck flexed (chin on the chest)

Puncture
— Puncture of the spinal canal, mostly at the L3/L4 level (or at L4/L5)
— Withdrawal of spinal fluid for cytological examination
— Contrast injection (injection speed 10 mL/60 sec)
— At the end of the injection, the needle is withdrawn, patient turned once completely around

Contrast media
— Intrathecal, 10 mL nonionic (Omnipaque 180)
— Intravenous, 100 mL nonionic (Omnipaque 300) as a bolus injection if there is a possibility of a tumor

Window algorithm
— Window level:
  40–60 HU (increased if the contrast is very dense)
— Window width:
  400–500 HU (up to 2000 HU if the contrast concentration is very dense)

Postoperative care
— Bed rest for 24 hrs
— Head strictly elevated (position of the rest of the body does not matter)
— Increased fluid intake (about 2–3 qts)

Tips & Tricks
— Take a scout view at each new scan level to facilitate postscan review at the different scan levels
— Identify and label the vertebral levels (L4, L5) or their corresponding intervertebral space (L4/L5)
— At the end, keep a survey film on hard copy of all the scans that were done

Abduction	Movement away from the body
Adduction	Movement toward the body
Anteflexion	Bending forward
Anterior	In front
Anterior-posterior (a.-p.)	From the front toward the back
Articulation	Joint
Boxer position	*see* LAO (second oblique diameter)
Bregmatic	Pertaining to the bregma (the junction between the coronal and sagittal sutures)
Cave	Beware
Caudal	Downwar
Caudocranial	From below to above
Caudodorsal	From below (obliquely) toward the back
Caudomedial	From below (obliquely) toward teh middle
Concave	Bending inward
Convex	Bending outward
Cranial	Upward
Craniocaudal	From above to below
Craniolateral	From above (Obliquely) to the side
Cranioventral	From above (obliquely) to the front
Diffuse radiation screen	Slats used to prevent diffuse radiation arising in the object
Distal	Away from (the center of) the body
Dorsal	Toward the back
Dorsoplantar	From the back of the foot to the sole
Dorsoventral (d.-v.)	From the back to the front
Dorsovolar	From the back of the hand to the palm
Expiration	Breathing out
Eye-ear line	The reference line between the lateral corner of the eye and the center of the auditory canal
Fencer position	*see* RAO (first oblique diameter)
FFD	Focus-film-distance
Fibular	Towards the calf
Frontal	Toward the forehead
German horizontal	The reference line between the lower edge of the eye and the upper external auditory canal
Gradual sheet	Compensation sheet
Gray	Unit of energy dosage (formerly rad; 1 rad = 0.01 Gy)
Humeroulnar	From the upper arm obliquely toward the ulna
Inclination	Bending forward
Inspiration	Breathing in
LAO	Left anterior oblique (front left oblique), second oblique diameter
Lateral	At the side
Laterodorsal	From the side (obliquely) toward the back
Lateroventral	From the side (obliquely) toward the front
Lordosis	Curvature of the spine toward the front
Medial	Toward the middle
Mediosagittal	In the center of the long axis of the body
Occipital	Toward the back of the head
Occipitomental	From the back of the head toward the chin

Occipitonasal	From the back of the head towards the nose
Occipito-orbital	From the back of the head toward the orbit (cavity containing the eyeball)
Palmar	Toward the palm of the hand
Philtrum	Median groove in the upper lip
Plantar	Toward the sole of the foot
Posterior	At the back
Posterior-anterior (p.-a.)	From the back toward the front
Pronation	Rotating inward
Proximal	Near the body, toward the middle of the body
Radial	Toward the radius
Radioulnar	From the radius toward the ulna
RAO	Right anterior oblique (front right oblique), second oblique diameter
Reclination	Bending backward
Retroflexion	*see* Reclination
Scoliosis	Curvature of the spine toward the side
Sensitivity class	Sensitivity of the film sheet system (sensitivity class 100 corresponds to a dosage requirement of 100 µGy for an optical density [D = l] higher than the veil or base)
Submental	Under the chin
Submentobregmatic	From the chin to the bregma (junction of the coronal and sagittal sutures)
Ulnar	Toward the ulna
Ulnohumeral	From the ulna (obliquely) toward the upper arm
Ulnoradial	From the ulna toward the radius
Ventral	Toward the abdomen
Ventrodorsal (v.-d.)	From the abdomen toward the back
Volar	Toward the Palm

Bernau A. Orthopädische Röntgendiagnostik—Einstelltechnik. Munich: Urban & Schwarzenberg; 1982

Brusis T, Mödder U. HNO-Röntgenaufnahmetechnik. Berlin: Springer; 1984.

Dietze R, Köcher E. Physik und Praxis der Röntgenaufnahmetechnik. Jena: Fischer; 1982.

Greenspan A. Atlas of Orthopedic Radiology. New York: Raven Press; 1992.

Hip E. Röntgendiagnostik. In: Witt AN et al. Orthopädie in Praxis und Klinik; vol 2. Stuttgart: Thieme 1980.

Hogarth B. Anatomisches Zeichnen leichtgemacht. Berlin: Taschen; 1991.

Husmann K, Mehrkens A, Hancken G. Radiologische Einstelltechnik. Berlin: Blackwell; 1995.

Jungbauer M. Röntgen-Einstelltechnik; vols. 1–4. Basel: Roche; 1979.

Leitlinien der Bundesärztekammer zu Qualitätssicherung in der Computertomographie. Dtsch Ärztebl. 1992; 89:49.

Lichte-Wichmann M. Richtig eingestellt? Stuttgart: Thieme; 1993.

Lutz K-Ch. Einstelltechniken in der Traumatologie. Stuttgart: Thieme; 1992.

Marcelis S, Seragini F, Taylor J, Huang G-S, Park Y-H, Resnick D. Cervical spine: comparison of 45° and 55° anteroposterior oblique radiographic projections. Radiology. 1993; 188:253–256.

Meschan I. Analyse der Röntgenbilder. Stuttgart: Enke; 1981.

Meschan I. Röntgenanatomie. Stuttgart: Enke; 1987.

Möller TB. Röntgennormalbefunde. Stuttgart: Thieme; 1987.

Möller TB, Klose K Ch. Rezeptbuch der Radiologie. Berlin: Springer; 1989.

Möller TB, Reif E. Taschenatlas der Röntgenanatomie. Stuttgart: Thieme; 1991.

Möller TB, Reif E. Taschenatlas der Schnittbildanatomie; vols 1, 2. Stuttgart: Thieme; 1993.

Oetjen H-W. Qualitätssicherung in der Computertomographie. Radiol Assist. 1994; H.2.

Poppe H. Technik der Röntgendiagnostik. 3rd ed. Stuttgart: Thieme; 1972.

Ring B. Felsenbeinaufnahme nach Mayer. Radiol Assist. 1991; H3.

Ring-Baltruweit B. Schädel in 2 Ebenen. Radiol Assist. 1993; H1.

Rubins DK. Anatomie für Künstler. Ravensburg, Germany: Maier; 1970.

Saß U. Qualitätskriterien röntgendiagnostischer Untersuchungen. Radiol Assist. 1991; H3.

Tertilt A. Schwedenstatus. Radiol Assist. 1990; H1.

Wandt C. Ala- und Obturatum-Aufnahme. Radiol Assist. 1992; H2.

Wandt C. Axiale oder axilläre Schultergelenk-Aufnahme. Radiol Assist. 1993; H3.

Wilhelm M. Vorschriftensammlung zum Vollzug der Röntgenverordnung. Munich: WRW-Verlags-GmbH; 1995.

Zimmer E A, Zimmer-Brossy M. Lehrbuch der röntgendiagnostischen Einstelltechnik. Berlin: Springer; 1982.

Index